TOWARDS BEST PRACTICES FOR SURVEYING PEOPLE WITH DISABILITIES

VOLUME 1

TOWARDS BEST PRACTICES FOR SURVEYING PEOPLE WITH DISABILITIES

VOLUME 1

THILO KROLL
DAVID KEER
PAUL PLACEK
JULIANA CYRIL
AND
GERRY HENDERSHOT
EDITORS

Nova Science Publishers, Inc.
New York

For permission to use material from this book please contact us:
Telephone 631-231-7269; Fax 631-231-8175
Web Site: http://www.novapublishers.com

Library of Congress Cataloging-in-Publication Data
Available upon request

ISBN 13: 978-1-60021-195-9
ISBN 10: 1-60021-195-X

Published by Nova Science Publishers, Inc. ✢ New York

CONTENTS

PREFACE

Thilo Kroll
University of Dundee, Scotland (UK)

In the United States 12.1 percent of the working age population between the ages of 21 and 64 have reported a disability in 2004. This estimate is based on the 2004 American Community Survey (ACS). In the same survey, physical disabilities constituted the largest group with 7.6% of the adult population in the aforementioned age group, followed by mental disabilities (4.2%) and sensory disabilities (2.8%) (Rehabilitation Research and Training Center on Disability Demographics and Statistics, 2005). There is further evidence that the number of people who report disabling conditions is on the increase, rising from 49 million during 1991-1992 to 54 million during 1994-1995 (MMWR, 2001). Estimates derived from the National Health Interview Survey (1983-1996) further indicate a significant increase in childhood disability rates (Fujiura and Kyoshi, 2000). Despite best efforts, there is significant concern among disability researchers that current data on disability do not tell the full story, and that survey research efforts may not be fully inclusive of people with various disabilities. Policy and program development depend on reliable data, and may run the risk of failing to improve the population's health well-being if they are based on skewed evidence.

It is the principal objective of the ***Disability and Health*** book series to provide a better understanding of the complex relationships between disability, health, and health care. ***Disability and Health*** specifically focuses on the intersection of disability, physical and social health. It features innovative conceptual reviews and reports as well as research articles. The scope of ***Disability and Health*** is international and multidisciplinary and it features the work from professionals of the various professional disciplines involved in health care, rehabilitation, and disability research.

The health focus in disability becomes increasingly important as people with various disabling conditions live longer and may experience an earlier onset of chronic health problems when compared to people without disabilities (Bauman et al., 1999; Campbell, Sheets and Strong, 1999).

This volume focuses on Best Practices for Surveying People with Disabilities. It is no coincidence that we focus on this topic at the beginning of this book series. The issue of accurate measurement in disability has concerned disability researchers for some time. Criticism has focused on the exclusion of critical disability groups from participation in national surveys because of a lack of alternative formats in the survey administration, inappropriate handling of proxy responses, insufficient interviewer training to accommodate people with disabilities, and undersampling.

It is of crucial importance to remedy the problem of survey exclusion of people with disabilities in order to arrive at correct estimates about the prevalence of disability to inform social and health policy.

Over the past three years The Washington Group on Disability Statistics has provided a new focus for measurement issues in the area of disability. It continued the activities that had begun at the United Nations International Seminar on Measurement of Disability that took place in New York on June 4-6, 2001. Participants included representatives from national statistical offices, disability measurement experts, representatives of the disability community, and other users of disability data.

More recently, in April 2004, the Interagency Committee on Disability Research hosted a two-day conference in Washington D.C. to specifically address the issue of survey practices in the field of disability. This book grew out of the presentations made at this meeting.

This book is primarily a book for researchers and practitioners in the disability field. Since the topics presented in the book crosscut multiple disciplines it may be suited for students and experts from various academic and professional backgrounds. It hopefully also finds many interested readers among students and teachers of medical, social and disability sciences at colleges and universities. While some chapters highlight the currently unresolved barriers towards obtaining accurate measurements for certain disability populations, others introduce innovative ways to plan for and to conduct inclusive surveys. In many instances, the work presented is work in progress and as such it is important in that it is expected to stimulate debate and future research work.

The chapters in this book focus on three central themes.

- Current Challenges in Survey Development for People with Disabilities
- Strategies to Promote Inclusion of People with Disabilities in Survey Development
- Issues for Future Development

This book combines the experience of survey researchers and administrators in the 'field' with a reflection on how survey methodology can be rendered more inclusive. The contributors to this volume discuss shortfalls of current survey methods and present innovative approaches to maximize inclusion of people with physical, sensory and psychiatric disabilities.

This volume of 'Disability and Health' has four accomplished disability researchers who have been instrumental in the debate about how to measure 'disability', 'health', and 'participation' accurately as co-editors.

Paul Placek, PhD who worked for more than 30 years as a senior scientist at the Centers for Disease Control, National Center for Health Statistics in Hyattsville, MD until his retirement in 2004. Dr. Placek has contributed significantly to conceptual debates and research in the area of disability classification, especially with regard to the WHO's International Classification of Functioning, Disability and Health (ICF).

David Keer, MA is a Program Specialist of the Research Sciences Division and a Co-Chair of the Interagency Subcommittee on Disability at the, National Institute on Disability and Rehabilitation Research, (NIDRR), Washington, DC, USA. For many years, he has been instrumental in promoting interagency communication about disability research and measurement issues.

Juliana Cyril, PhD is a Scientific Program Administrator at the Office of Public Health Research at the Centers for Disease Control and Prevention in Atlanta, GA. Dr. Cyril's work has focused on disability measurement topics across the life span.

Gerry Hendershot, PhD is a consultant for disability and health statistics. Until 2003, he worked as a senior scientist at the Centers for Disease Control and Prevention, National Center for Health Statistics where he was one of the authors of the National Health Interview Survey (NHIS).

ACKNOWLEDGEMENTS

The editors would like to thank Barbara Rosen of Cherry Engineering Support Services, Inc (CESSI) for her help to organize the conference that led to this volume. Also, we like to express our gratitude to the authors who contributed to this valuable volume.

REFERENCES

Bauman, W.A,, Adkins, R.A., Spungen, A.M. and R.L. Waters (1999). The Effect of Residual Neurological Deficit on Oral Glucose Tolerance in Persons with Chronic Spinal Cord Injury. *Spinal Cord*, 37(11), 765-771.

Campbell, M.L., Sheets, D. and Strong, P.S. (1999). Secondary health conditions among middle-aged individuals with chronic physical disabilities: implications for unmet needs for services. *Assistive Technology,* 11(2),105-22.

Fujiura, G.T. and Yamaki, K. (2000). Trends in childhood disability prevalence: Poverty and family structure. *Exceptional Children*, 66, 187-199.

Rehabilitation Research and Training Center on Disability Demographics and Statistics (2005). *2004 Disability Status Reports*. Ithaca, NY: Cornell University.

Prevalence of Disabilities and Associated Health Conditions Among Adults in the United States, 1999. *MMWR* 50(7), 2001.

BEST PRACTICES FOR SURVEYING PEOPLE WITH DISABILITIES: AN INTRODUCTION

David Keer[1]
National Institute on Disability and Rehabilitation Research (NIDRR),
U.S. Department of Education

INTRODUCTION

The Interagency Committee on Disability Research (ICDR) promotes coordination and cooperation among Federal departments and agencies conducting rehabilitation research programs. In April 2004, the ICDR's Interagency Subcommittee on Disability Statistics (ISDS) sponsored a two-day conference on "Best Practices for Surveying People with Disabilities." Almost 100 individuals from the federal sector, private organizations, and universities, discussed enhancements in survey design and methodology to maximize inclusion of respondents with disabilities in national surveys. Several researchers and practitioners who had presented research at the conference contributed the papers in this volume.

Full inclusion of people with disabilities in surveys provides useful and accurate information for research, policymaking, and advocacy. Barriers to inclusion can occur at many stages of the survey process. As noted throughout this volume, use of a participatory action research (PAR) approach is a good starting point to avoid methodological problems. Consumer advisors bring a focus that can assure that a survey includes the right questions asked of the right people in the right way. PAR in the survey context requires time and cooperation but strengthens relevance and quality.

Several authors describe implementation of PAR in the survey context. Jonathan Delman is the founder of Consumer Quality Initiatives, a mental health, consumer-staffed and directed

---

[1] The views expressed herein do not necessarily represent the positions or policies of the U.S. Department of Education or member agencies of the ICDR. No official endorsement by the U.S. Department of Education, or any ICDR member agency, of any product, commodity, service or enterprise mentioned in this publication is intended or should be inferred.

research organization. In "**Consumer-Driven and Conducted Survey Research in Action**", Delman describes a community-based, participatory action research model that brings consumers into all aspects of the research process. Consumers determine program outcome priorities to measure, conduct interviews, and write reports with recommendations to improve quality in the mental health system. Consumers-as-interviewers can help establish rapport among disenfranchised individuals with disabilities. The work of Consumer Quality Initiatives demonstrates that appropriate accommodations and supports enable people with mental illness to conduct significant research activities.

Alexis Henry, Patricia Gallagher, Vickie Stringfellow, Leslie Olin Fred Hooven, and Jay Himmelstein report on a survey conducted under the Massachusetts Medicaid Infrastructure Grant (MMIG) involving multiple stakeholders (**"Contemporary Strategies for Developing Surveys of People with Disabilities: The MassHealth Employment and Disability Survey"**). The survey yielded information relevant to the goals of the MMIG and to stakeholders. Henry's group also employed a participatory action research (PAR) approach that included stakeholders as active members of the research team. True PAR requires stakeholder involvement from the initial study design through interpretation and presentation of results and the formulation of action steps. Power sharing, informed decision making and continued involvement of stakeholders in the process may be challenges to more traditional approaches.

"Using American Sign Language in Assessing the End-of-Life-Care Educational Needs of Deaf Persons" from Barbara Allen, Nancy Meyers, John Sullivan, and Melissa Sullivan Allen describes research to assess the needs of deaf seniors for information about health care and legal issues related to end-of-life care. Steps in the process included individual and focus group interviews with representatives of the deaf community to evaluate and revise the questionnaire. Deaf interviewers used ASL-GLOSS, an American Sign Language linguistic method, to interview deaf respondents who were dependent on signed language. Following the interviews, the project included a multistage process in which deaf interviewers coded both the closed-ended and open-ended survey questions. In tandem with community leaders and hearing researchers the interviewers also reviewed and interpreted the findings.

The Allen report provides a nice overview of a community-based participatory research (CBPR) strategy. It is good reading for researchers less familiar with CBPR. Beyond that, the paper includes a discussion of specific issues in design of questionnaires for deaf respondents. All survey practitioners will benefit from that discussion. Overall, the innovations in survey design and method that are described had a significant impact on collecting valid and reliable data. Some of the lessons may have value in surveys of other linguistic minority populations.

As noted by the American Association for Public Opinion Research, one must "take great care in matching question wording to the concepts being measured and the population studied."[2] Mitchell LaPlante, Stephen Kaye, Joseph Mullan, and Alice Wong from the Disability Statistics Center at the UCSF, work to improve the ability of national surveys to more validly identify people with disabilities with a short set of questions. In "**Initial Development of the Disability & Activity Impact Screener (DAIS): An Example of Qualitative Measurement Discovery**," LaPlante starts with the premise that people with

---

[2] American Association for Public Opinion Research. (2002). *Best Practices for Survey and Public Opinion Research.* Lenexa, KS.

disabilities must endorse the questions concerning disability on surveys. Here and elsewhere in his portfolio of work, LaPlante has observed a disconnect between the lived experience of respondents and questions which are driven by medical and functional models. That disconnect raises concerns about the validity and reliability of some existing measures.

LaPlante and his colleagues conducted focus groups with participants who discussed disability in their daily lives, including definitions of disability, physical barriers and challenging situations. Independent researchers coded the data from the groups and identified common themes. Notably, problematic social interactions, management strategies, and the idea that people with disabilities do things differently captured many of the conversations. Based on these themes, LaPlante's group developed Disability Activity Impact Screener (DAIS).

During subsequent cognitive testing, people with disabilities endorsed the new question set. Interviewees indicated that they could understand the new questions and that the questions were a more accurate reflection of their disability experience. LaPlante recommends including people with disabilities from the start of instrument development as a method to improve future surveys. Strategies such as focus groups and cognitive interviews are known tools for improving survey questions. LaPlante's work, similar to that of Delman's and Henry's groups, demonstrates the strength of strong consumer participation from the earliest stages of conceptual design.

Stephen Kaye from the University of California at San Francisco's (UCSF) Disability Statistics Center and Center for Personal Assistance Services analyzed response patterns in the National Health Interview Survey (NHIS) and the NHIS on Disability (NHIS-D). The NHIS-D was a two-stage survey conducted from 1994-1997 with household screening during Phase I and individual interviews with individuals with disabilities during Phase II. As noted in "**Inclusion of People with Disabilities in the NHIS and NHIS-D: Non-response, Proxy-response, and Assisted Response,**" the National Center for Health Statistics (NCHS) strove to maximize self-response during the Phase II. NCHS had developed video and other training materials to teach interviewers how to interview people with disabilities.

Careful planning resulted in a high self-response rate during Phase II. Not all disability groups, however, were well represented. Persons with a greater need for assistance with activities of daily living had substantially lower self-response rates than other persons with disabilities. People with cognitive disabilities rarely respond for themselves. Those persons who were deaf or who had speech impairments also had low rates of self-response. On the other hand, self-response was good among people with mental health disabilities or with mobility or visual impairments.

Using data from the 1997 and later National Health Interview Survey, Kaye also discusses impact of changes in self-response rules on non-response among individuals with cognitive and severe physical disabilities. Kaye's findings demonstrate that self-response, assisted response, and proxy response can help assure collection of data about individuals with all types of disabilities. As Kaye recommends, better accommodations help ensure the full participation of people with all types of disabilities in national surveys.

In "**Removing the Barriers: Modifying Telephone Survey Methodology to Increase Self-Response Among People with Disabilities,**" Anne Ciemnecki and Karen CyBulski also address the necessity for collecting information directly from respondents with disabilities. Ciemnecki and CyBulski tackle the need to assure that a telephone survey is accessible to all respondents. As they note, telephone surveys are a cost-effective way to collect data. To maximize inclusion via that method, the researcher must address challenges raised by:

- Communication difficulties such as speech and hearing impairments;
- Stamina problems including physical and mental fatigue; and
- Cognitive issues ranging from emotional disturbance to difficulty processing questions to not having the knowledge to answer the questions and confusion about the interview.

Ciemnicki and CyBulski developed a toolkit of modifications for survey design. Modifications included shorter interviews, rest breaks during the interview, minimizing high frequency sounds, checkpoints, and structured probes. The strategies to maximize self-response are neither difficult to implement nor costly. Many of the techniques benefit both individuals with and without disabilities. Similar to Kaye's work, this paper notes that self-responders often provide more complete information than proxy respondents.

Kristine Mulhorn's "**Addressing Recommendations for Increasing Rate of Response by Persons with Disabilities**," draws upon work of the international research team DISTAB (Disability Tabulations), which began operation in 1999 as a continuation of the United Nations' project DISTAT. DISTAB members created "quality profiles," which inventory key methodological features of six nationally representative health surveys that include disability questions. The surveys, one from each of six different countries, allow international comparison of sample size and methods of data collection. The United States' National Health Interview Survey on Disability was one of the six surveys.

Mulhorn cites recommendations from the National Council on Disability (NCD) for conducting disability research. NCD has long advocated participation of individuals with disabilities in the research process. Using the NCD framework, DISTAB identified a number of practices for involving people with disabilities in the survey process. Across the six surveys, a variety of approaches to the stages of the survey process - from questionnaire design through sampling plan, data collection, and analysis,- suggest the need for flexibility and creativity. Organizations that support people with disabilities can be resources to assure appropriate survey design and outputs.

Patrick Murray, from Rutgers University's Eagleton Institute, discusses a case study that examined options for conducting a self-administered survey among the blind and visually impaired. "**A Multi-Mode Approach for Surveying Visually Impaired Populations**," reports on a state-funded survey that was conducted for the New Jersey Commission for the Blind and Visually Impaired in 1997 and again in 2003. In 1997, respondents had the option of completing the survey in one of several modes: a large print version, by Braille, by computer disk or by audio tape, and one interview-assisted mode by calling a staffed toll-free telephone number. Because of budget constraints the 2003 survey did not include options for Braille, audio tape, or computer disk. In both years, the researchers used the same questionnaire and a three-wave mail design.

The budgetary constraints created an opportunity to consider the question of impact of multiple modes on both response rate and the representative nature of the data itself. During 1997, about 70 percent of clients who responded completed the survey by mail using large print format with almost all the other respondents completing the survey via telephone. Only nine of the 525 respondents requested Braille, audiotape, or computer disk. In 2003, the telephone option again increased response rate. The survey across the two years suggests that accessibility and budget can be balanced to maximize participation by individuals with disabilities. Murray's research underscores the need for additional studies to evaluate the impact of multiple modes of data collection across different disability populations.

A newer approach to facilitating access is through technology and the Internet. One example is provided by Judith Cook, Genevieve Fitzgibbon, Drew Batteiger, and Dennis D. Grey from the University of Illinois at Chicago. "**Results of a Web Survey of Self-Determination Among Individuals with Psychiatric Disabilities Who Do and Do Not Receive Mental Health Services** reports on research to gather data from mental health consumers about their experiences related to self-determination, the service delivery system and uses of information technology. Individuals with psychiatric disabilities are often reluctant to disclose their disability. The Internet survey provides greater anonymity that could increase response and data quality.

Cook's survey drew upon items from the Pew Internet Life Project, the Census Technology Project, and the April 2003 Pew Project report on "Internet Access and the Digital Divide." A participatory action workgroup was used to adapt the individual survey items. An outside vendor provided the software for survey development software and for Web survey hosting and data collection. The sample was obtained through mental health listservs, Web sites, mailings and newsletter advertising.

One must balance the advantages of a web-based survey against some clear limitations. The sample itself is limited by issues of self-selection and access to the Internet. Ideally, a web-based survey could be used in conjunction with other strategies for data collection. In the absence of a multi-pronged approach to data collection, results form the web-based survey must be interpreted cautiously.

Nonetheless, for some populations the Internet strategy may provide a comfort level that allows for participation.

"**How to Reach the Invisible Population of Hard of Hearing Adults in Main Street America**," by John Schroedel, offers a perspective on the key issue of sampling. Identifying a frame for sampling the population of individuals with disabilities is a difficult task. For specific populations, such as individuals with hearing loss, the costs can be high. As a result, much research about this population relies on convenience samples from consumer or related organizations. Schroedel relied on developing a national sample by telephone screening. He then conducted a follow-up survey via mail.

Schroedel's work underscores a pressing need for research to improve sampling strategies that capture individuals with disabilities, especially disabilities which are harder to identify or which occur less frequently. The National Health Interview Survey on Disability in 1994 – 1995 used an extensive battery of questions to identify the sample for a followback survey. The costs of that approach are unwieldy for most survey research.

Ray Glazier from Abt Associates describes an approach to "**Training Temporarily Able-Bodied Survey Interviewers**," Glazier's paper is a good resource for those who work in field operations. Glazier's guide illustrates that there is not a one-size-fits-all strategy for data collection among individuals with disabilities. The many specific pointers for interviewers can facilitate a successful survey.

As a group, the papers provide a good foundation for improving survey practice to maximize inclusion of people with disabilities. First and foremost, participatory action research offers many advantages in the survey design and implementation process.

Individuals with disabilities can provide insights to help assure that the questions being asked yield useful information, can identify the need for accommodations in the interview process, and are often the most sensitive and effective interviewers. As a general rule, a universal design research strategy is a gold standard to improve accessibility of surveys and quality of data.

Existing tools such as cognitive interviews and field testing are fundamental for development of measures appropriate to specific disability populations. Individuals with cognitive disabilities and those who are deaf and hard of hearing may merit increased attention during the testing process. In general, as with any survey, consumer-consultants can assist in assuring question order placement that achieves the goals of the survey and simplifies the task for the respondent.

Sample design may pose particular challenges. Individuals with disabilities from diverse populations or with less common impairments or functional limitations

pose unique challenges for representation in surveys. Depending upon the research goals, it may be necessary to over sample for sub-populations. The screening questions are especially important in this regard. In some situations, one might be able to compensate for small populations during analysis.

The mode of data collection may impact survey participation for individuals with disabilities. Telephone, mail, face-to-face, and web-based surveys each has pros and cons for specific disability groups. In some cases, as discussed in these papers, potential limitations can be addressed with simple modification. In the best case scenario a multimodal survey could address the needs of diverse disability groups. A caveat is the need to assess the impact of multiple modes on understanding of, and response to, the survey questions.

Though generally preferred, there may be occasions when self-response is not a reasonable option. Assisted response is an alternative that can be respectful of individuals with disabilities. For some surveys, proxy response is preferable to no response. Accommodations such as breaks in the interview might allow respondents to self-respond over a period of two or three sittings. Simplified question wording could enable others to respond for themselves. Interviewer training must address criteria for moving away from self-response.

Rest breaks can be an important accommodation for respondents. Interviewers must not be penalized for recognizing the need to pause the interview. It may be the case that, to allow full participation by respondents with disabilities, the survey enterprise must revisit demands upon the interviewer to achieve production targets. In tandem with additional interviewer training, this is an area of enhancement that will have an impact on survey costs. Over time, organizations may develop a corps of interviewers with necessary expertise.

It is worth noting that building accommodations into the survey process would benefit respondents both with and without disabilities. As the population ages, it is increasingly helpful for the principles of universal design to be incorporated into surveys. Vision and hearing difficulties are not restricted to individuals with the label "disability". Many respondents could benefit from a break during a lengthy interview. Interviewers themselves might find accommodations helpful. With the following papers as a starting point, it remains to continue research into accessible and affordable methodologies.

In: Towards Best Practices for Surveying People..., Volume 1 ISBN 1-60021-195-X
Editors: Thilo Kroll, David Keer et al., pp. 1-11

Chapter 1

ADDRESSING RECOMMENDATIONS FOR INCREASING THE RATE OF RESPONSE BY PERSONS WITH DISABILITIES: A COMPARISON ACROSS SIX NATIONAL SURVEYS

Kristine A. Mulhorn[1]
Associate Professor,Department of Health Sciences and Administration
University of Michigan-Flint,303 E. Kearsley St.Flint, MI 48502

ABSTRACT

This chapter summarizes the efforts in six countries to increase the response rate of persons with disabilities in their national disability surveys. The strategies presented by the members of DISTAB (*DIS*ability *TAB*ulations)—a group sponsored by the National Center for Health Statistics to examine cross-national comparability of disability statistics—present a set of recommendations for future surveys. The countries included in DISTAB are Australia, Canada, France, The Netherlands, South Africa and the United States. Each country's disability survey is described according to basic information such as methodological aspects, time frame, response rate and sample size. The description of the strategies for increasing the response rate of persons with disabilities follows an outline of topics described by the National Council on Disability in 1998. The topics include 1) choosing topics, objectives, and variables; 2) choosing methods of data collection; 3) designing the sample; 4) designing the questionnaire; 5) collecting the data; and 6) analyzing and reporting the data. These topics were summarized into five questions that can be considered in the development of disability surveys, and for each of these questions, examples from the participating countries are described. For example, almost all of the countries used specific strategies to involve persons with disabilities in the planning or developing of the survey. The questions and the answers to them for each survey make up what is called a quality profile. These questions can be asked for all disability surveys, providing the start of a "gold standard" for conducting disability surveys.

---

[1] email: kmulhorn@umflint.edu

INTRODUCTION

Disability surveillance at the national level is a standard practice in many countries. But comparing disability statistics across countries continues to present stumbling blocks. In one effort to move toward strategies for comparing disability rates across countries, members of an international research team called the DISTAB group have developed a recommended strategy for improving survey research by increasing the representativeness of persons with disabilities.

BACKGROUND

The purpose of this paper is to describe one strategy for comparing methodological issues in disability surveys and, as a result, move toward a "gold standard" of methodological practices for all national surveys.

The DISTAB (*DIS*ability*TAB*ulations) Group is an international team of survey statisticians representing national disability surveys in six countries (Greenberg and Heick, 2002).. The group was sponsored by the National Center for Health Statistics and led by Dr. Paul Placek, Senior Statistician, in an effort to address the comparability of disability statistics and to assist in the testing and the development of the International Classification of Functioning, Disability and Health (ICF) (WHO, 2001). The first meeting was in 1999, and at that time the participating countries were Canada, France, Netherlands, South Africa and the US. Later, Australia joined as a permanent member. A related purpose of the group was to compare rates of disability across countries using the ICF as a conceptual framework.

While an in-depth discussion of the role of ICF in the comparability of these surveys was reported in an earlier paper (Swanson, Carrothers, and Mulhorn, 2001), the current discussion addresses additional methodological aspects specifically for removing barriers to participation for persons with disabilities. Strengths and shortcomings of major national disability surveys from the DISTAB project are used to demonstrate this unique contribution to survey methodology.

DISTAB began several projects that attempted to compare the methodology used and the disability statistics produced by each country's national survey. To address the issue of removing barriers to inclusion of persons with disabilities, the group compared methodological approaches used to develop the surveys and to increase participation in the survey process. The comparison of the methodological approaches was influenced by an earlier report and subsequent work by Gerry Hendershot.

In 1998 the National Council on Disability (1998), the Federal ombudsman for people with disabilities, issued a report on "Reorienting Disability Research" that indicted the research community, including the survey community, for inhibiting the participation of PWD's at all stages of the research process (Hendershot, 1998). It is worth quoting some of the Council's recommendations as they relate to the stages of survey research.

1) *Choosing topics, objectives, and variables*: "Establish focus groups on the emerging issues and needs of persons with disabilities in the topical areas of major surveys before data collection instruments are planned. It is not enough to have people

review completed surveys; key constituencies must also be involved in defining the purpose and research questions of a study."

2) *Choosing methods of data collection*: "Methods needed to ensure everyone's participation in research depend on the specific research techniques used for most of the sample; for example, a telephone survey needs to accommodate direct participation by people with hearing and speech impairments."
3) *Designing the sample:* "Ensure that the broadest range of people with disabilities (including children, those with hidden disabilities, and minorities with disabilities) are sampled. To understand the unique aspects of all people with disabilities, it is critical that all groups be adequately sampled.
4) *Designing the questionnaire:* "Design well-written questions to measure work disability that separate the notions of employment and disability. Work limitations must be described in the data, not by inference, as a function of environmental barriers and accommodation, including transportation, along with individual impairment."
5) *Collecting the data:* "Information should be available in accessible formats in all phases of data collection activities."
6) *Analyzing and reporting the data:* "Ensure that data and data analyses are disseminated in alternative formats and that they are accessible to people with all disabilities. Formats such as Braille, large print, and computer disks will enable blind and visually impaired people to participate in all phases of disability research. Particular attention should be given to presentation of quantitative data commonly formatted in tables, graphs, and so on" (Hendershot, 1998). These six questions framed the questions in DISTAB's quality profiles so that the various measures used to increase participation among PWD's could be compared across the six countries.

Methods

"Quality profiles" are inventories of the methodological aspects of surveys. Some of these methodological aspects include sample size, response rate, data collection period, and data collection methodology (Office of Management and Budget, 2001). The DISTAB group enhanced this concept by focusing on the unique methodological aspects of disability surveys. Five questions specifically addressing the inclusion of PWD's were added to the quality profiles used by the DISTAB group. The quality profiles then became the means for comparison. The next section includes descriptions of each of the surveys and the results section displays the quality profile contents for each of these five questions. One limitation of the study is that it represents results from six countries and is not representative of countries in the developing world.

The disability survey quality profiles suggested here were first identified by Gerry Hendershot, former Branch Chief in charge of analysis of the Health Interview Survey at the National Center for Health Statistics. He summarized recommendations for removing barriers to survey participation for persons with disabilities (Hendershot, 2003). He suggested that a paradigm shift is needed in survey research. He argued that there are areas in survey development and the analysis process where barriers should be removed and persons with disabilities should be involved. Based on the questions stated earlier from the NCD report, these are: choosing topics, objectives and variables as the survey is being developed; choosing methods of data collection; designing the sample; designing the questionnaire; collecting the data; analyzing and reporting the data. We suggest that these five questions should be added to the standard methodological quality profiles so that each country can outline specific procedures to encourage response by PWD's These questions are: 1) Were PWD's involved in planning or developing the survey? 2) Were sampling strategies implemented to increase representativeness of PWD's (e.g., screening)? 3) Was the survey instrument produced in multiple formats to accommodate PWD's (e.g., TTY, large type)? 4) What efforts were made to produce the results in multiple formats for dissemination? 5) Were questions asked to elicit information about environment and/or participation? This last question combines two stages of survey development—the administration of the survey and the dissemination of the survey.

SURVEY DESCRIPTIONS

Descriptions of existing national surveys of the participating countries are given below All are nationally-representative health surveys with questions focusing on disability. The descriptions were provided by members of the DISTAB group, which met annually, face-to-face, and monthly international telephone conference calls to accomplish its goals.

Australia: Survey of Disability, Ageing And Carers

Last conducted in 2003, the Survey of Disability, Ageing and Carers is the principle source of information on people with disabilities, older persons, and those who provide care to people because of their disability. It collects information on three population groups: people aged 60 and over, people with disabilities and their caregivers. There are other sources of information about services provided to these groups, but this survey is the only source of information on the assistance requirements of those groups, the extent to which these requirements are met, and the characteristics of those with unmet need. It also provides information on participation in economic and community activities. The survey is the major source of national statistics on caregivers and primary caregivers, the numbers and characteristics of caregivers, care relationships, activities for which informal care is provided, and, for primary caregivers, support available and the effects of the caregiving role on their lives.

The data gathered for this survey are needed for policy development review, service planning and implementation, and general research. The size and distribution of groups eligible for assistance under different program legislation is used by the Commonwealth Departments of Health and Ageing, and Family and community Services as the basis for allocating and distributing program funds to State governments, and by State and Territory departments for service planning and fund distribution. The User Advisory Group which advised survey development included representatives from all levels of government, service providers, people with disabilities and academics.

All persons, of all ages in both private dwellings and institutions were eligible for inclusion with the following exceptions: overseas visitors (usually resident outside Australia); members of non-Australian defense forces (and their dependents); non-Australian diplomats (including diplomatic staff and non-Australian members of their household; inmates of reformatories; people in sparse and indigenous strata in the Northern Territory.

The survey has two components: the Household component and the Cared.

Accommodation Component

The Household component includes usual residents of private dwellings excluding those who had been away or were likely to be away for three months and residents of special dwellings (other than Health Establishments) who had been or were likely to be there for three months. The Cared accommodation component includes usual residents of selected Health Establishments who had been or were likely to be there for three months. An area sample of private dwellings, covering both urban and rural areas in all States and Territories (except for those living in remote and sparsely settled parts of Australia) was used. The list of non-private dwellings from the census was used to identify selected special dwellings (i.e., hospitals, nursing homes, retirement villages, homes for the aged, children's homes, and aged care hostels) to be sampled in the cared accommodation component of the survey. Most other non-private dwellings (e.g.,hotels, motels, and guesthouses) were also included in the household component. After exclusions due to scope and coverage, the final sample comprised 36,951 persons for the household component and 5,716 persons for the cared accommodation component. The calculation of non-response rates had the following results: 83.8% fully responded; 9.3% gave partial non-responses (mainly income questions); 6.9% provided what were identified as full non-responses; only 1.8% refused; for 3% there was no contact and 2.1% were classified as "other". For the Cared accommodation component, 93.4% fully responded to the questions.

Canada: Health and Activity Limitation Survey (HALS) 1991

The Health and Activity Limitation Survey (HALS) was designed to collect data for a national database on disability (Statistics Canada, 1991). HALS was first conducted after the 1986 Census of Population and repeated after the 1991 Census of Population. HALS collects data on: the nature and severity of disabilities; the barriers that persons with disabilities face in household tasks, employment, education, accommodation, transportation, finances, and recreation and lifestyles; the use of and need for assistive devices; and the out-of-pocket expenses related to disability. HALS consists of two separate components: the Household Survey, conducted immediately following the 1991 census and the Institutions Survey, conducted in early 1992. The sample size for the household survey was 148,000 and the sample size for the institutions Survey was 10,000 persons. The response rate for the household survey was 87% and the response rate for the institutions survey in 1991 was 96% (Statistics Canada, 1991).

France: France Handicaps-Disabilities-Dependency Survey (HID)

HID was the first French survey which attempts to achieve a national comprehensive coverage of all types of disabilities of every level of severity (formal registration or self recognition) of people of all ages, living in institutional settings and households (INSEE, 1999). This survey has been conducted by INSEE (Institut national de la statistique et des études économiques) with the support of a scientific committee that had expertise in statistics, disability research, and public administration. HID had two components: the household survey and the institutions survey, conducted by questionnaire. The institutional settings have been surveyed twice, in 1998 and 2000 (INSEE, 1999). The household survey was conducted in 1999 and in 2001. HID-Household was based on a sample of 20,116 households (or 21,760 persons) selected by means of a screening questionnaire applied on a representative sample of the national census of 1999 (this included 20 questions on health status). The response rates were 79.5% for households and 78% for institutionalized persons. The French data provided for DISTAB are drawn from the 1999 household survey. HID collected data on: 1) nature and origin of disability; 2) description of disability; 3) family and social environment; 4) technical aids and home adapted equipment used or needed; 5) housing conditions; 6) use of transportation; 7) education; 8) higher education; 9) financial resources and social security status; 10) leisure time, vacations and culture; 11) principal unpaid caregiver. One of the main aims of HID was to provide "gold standards" for prevalence and incidence rates of disability in France independently from the public system of disability support and benefits (INSEE, 1999).

Netherlands: Netherlands Health Interview Survey

Data for the calculation were derived from the combined Health Interview Surveys 1997 and 1998 in the Netherlands (Statistics Netherlands, 1996). The total N = 20,221, of which 14,899 respondents were age 18 years or older (Statistics Netherlands, 1996). Because in the Netherlands non-response in this type of survey is around 40%, a weighting factor for each individual respondent is calculated to make the sample representative of the Netherlands population. In short, this weighting factor is based on complete correspondence between distribution of (combinations of) sample- characteristics and known distributions of these characteristics in the total population: sex, age, marital status, municipality-status, province, household-size. Because the sample for Netherlands' Survey was drawn from a so-called container sample with known information, more information could be used for the weighting factors: labor force participation, perceived health and smoking behavior. The weighting factor is calculated in such a way that the weighted sample size is equal to the total Netherlands population (Statistics Netherlands, 1996).

South Africa:Baseline Survey On Disability

Data were collected in 1998 and represent responses from over 9,000 households and information on over 42,000 people of all ages (Schneider; Claassens.; Kimmie; Morgan; Naicker; Roberts.; McLaren,1999). The sample was a population-based representative sample stratified by province (9 in South Africa), rural, urban and metropolitan areas and race (Black, Colored, Indian and White). The interviews were carried out face-to-face in the language of the respondent's choice. Two questionnaires were administered. Every household was administered a screening questionnaire that determined whether a household had a disabled member or not. If there was a disabled person, the detailed questionnaire was administered to that person or their proxy. Around 2,300 people were identified as being disabled and of these, 1,703 were respondents to the detailed questionnaire. Questions about education, living arrangements and marital status were only asked of the sample of 1,703. The data are adjusted for age based on the 1996 South African census data. The domains of functioning covered included body movement, ADLs, seeing, mobility, learning, emotional, intellectual , hearing and speaking (Schneider, et al., 1999).

United States: The National Health Interview Survey on Disability (1994-95)

The National Health Interview Survey on Disability (NHIS-D) was a household survey of the non-institutionalized civilian population conducted in person by interviews by the the National Center for Health Statistics (Benson and Marano, 1998; NCHS, 1999a; NCHS, 1999b). This survey was conducted in two phases as a supplement to the annual National Health Interview Survey. NHIS-D, Phase I (1994 and 1995) was conducted concurrently with the core questionnaire and collected disability information for all members of the household. The questionnaire included basic questions about disability and was used as a screening device for a follow-up survey, NHIS-D Phase II. The 1994 NHIS-D Phase I included 107,469 persons and the 1995 NHIS-D Phase I included 95,091 persons. The total combined response rate was 87% for both years. The combined sample size used in this analysis was 145,007 adults (aged 18+ years) (NCHS, 1999a; NCHS, 1999b).

RESULTS

The following tables display methodological aspects of surveys used in the DISTAB surveys to encourage participation and response by PWD's. The tables are presented so that each table represents one of the five questions given above. All of the entries in the tables are recommendations for other survey researchers. Table 1 shows the results for the question, "Were persons with disabilities involved in planning or developing the survey? Five of the countries implemented some strategies. Cognitive testing was completed only in the US survey. Cognitive testing addresses how the questions are understood by the respondents and provides insight for wording, colloquial understandings of terms and other dimensions of survey questions that cannot be determined by other pre-testing methods. Two countries-- Australia and South Africa-- employed an advisory group or committee that was not part of the government organization designing the survey to advise on the content of the survey. In the US, persons with disabilities in one community were identified in advance through local agencies to be part of the design process. In addition to cognitive testing, the NCHS used mock interviews, and "dress rehearsals" with persons with disabilities to recommend and revise before the actual survey was carried out. Cognitive testing along with other methods such as pre-testing and observational studies were outlined as key strategies in the testing of surveys at the Workshop on Improving Disability Data for Policy Use in 2003 (Hillerman, 2003).

Table 1: Were persons with disabilities involved in planning or developing the survey?

US	cognitive testing; mock interviews, convenience samples to test; "dress rehearsals"; to ensure representativeness, PWD's in one community were identified in advance through local agencies
Canada	development of survey content, operations
Australia	extensive liaison with a user advisory group
France	design, development of survey content and testing
South Africa	work with ongoing committee that commented and advised throughout the process

Table 2 displays the sampling strategies implemented to increase representativeness of persons with disabilities. While the census is often used in the developing world as the source of disability information when a separate disability survey is not feasible, in some developed countries the census acts as a screening mechanism to determine if those individuals should be interviewed again for more detailed information. In the DISTAB countries, there was some form of screening implemented by three of the countries—Canada, France and the US. In Canada, there were filter questions on the survey to identify where follow-up could occur and there were screening questions on the survey itself. France used sampling based on additional survey questions added to the census that specifically addressed disability. While Canada's approach of using filter questions in the census and then returning to those households specifically identified by disability status, the approach used in the US was to apply two waves of a disability survey, which was integrated into the annual health interview survey. Then, in a second phase, those households identified as persons with disabilities were re-interviewed. Australia's approach was unique among the six countries because they created a shorter list of survey questions from which comparisons could be made between the populations with disabilities and those without. They also included two types of living arrangements to increase the representativeness of persons with disabilities. Both non-private dwellings (e.g., hotels, motels, and guest houses) and institutional accommodations were included among the survey respondents.

Table 2: Were the sampling strategies implemented to increase representativeness of PWD (e.g., screening)?

Canada	Filter questions on the census AND screening questions in the survey
France	Sampling based on the census AND screening
US	PWD populations were re-interviewed in the 2nd phase
Australia	Shorter set of questions for comparing PWD and those with no reported; inclusion of non-private dwellings (hotels/motels/guest houses; inclusion of institutionalized settings)

The third question asked was, "Was the instrument produced in multiple formats to accommodate PWD's (e.g., TTY, large type)?" In the administration of the survey, several alternative formats were used. Canada and South Africa used sign language interpreters as part of the surveying strategy. France presented the objectives of the survey in Synthetic Braille format. In the US, interviewers were allowed to use in-house interpreters, and some deaf persons received help with translation from others in the household.

Table 3: Was the survey instrument produced in multiple formats to accommodate PWD (e.g., TTY, large type)?

Canada, South Africa	sign language interpreters
France	synthetic Braille presentation of objectives of survey
US	interviewers were allowed to use in-house interpreters; some deaf persons had persons to help with translation

The answers to the fourth question are displayed in Table 4. The question was "Were the results produced in multiple formats to accommodate PWD's?" In the reporting of the results, again, multiple formats were applied. Australia and the US produced the results on CD-rom. In addition to the CD-rom format, Australia made the results available in various text formats. In Canada, some of the results were available Braille and audio formats. The Netherlands made the results available in multiple formats for download. Also, feedback workshops which included members of organizations of persons with disabilities provided additional communication about the results of the survey.

Table 4: Were the results produced in multiple formats to accommodate PWD's?

Australia	CD-Rom; also available in various text formats
Canada	some output in alternative format (Braille, audio)
Netherlands	multiple formats available for download; feedback workshops including some disabled persons organizations

The last two questions were questions asked to elicit information about the environment and / or participation. The results are combined and displayed in a grid (Table 5) with the countries representing the rows and topic areas representing environment and/or participation in the columns. There are multiple ways to define participation and environment. The topics applied in the DISTAB surveys include health services, education, employment (education and employment being important participation areas), social and/or leisure activities, housing, personal assistance, the built environment, and technical assistance (such as technical aids and transportation). These topics can be added to surveys about disability to demonstrate recognition of disability as a complex concept includes the role of participation and environment (WHO, 2001; Fougeryrollas and Beauregard, 2001).

Table 5. Were questions asked to elicit information about environment and/or participation?

.	Health Services	Education	Employment	Social/Leisure	Activities	Housing	Personal Assistant Built	Environment Techn	Assist.Aids Transportation	Additional Modules
Australia		✓	✓	✓		✓		✓	✓	
Canada		✓	✓	✓						
France		✓	✓	✓	✓	✓		✓		
Netherlands										✓
S. Aftrica		✓	✓				✓			
US	✓	✓	✓	✓		✓	✓	✓	✓	

Conclusions

The DISTAB group's work can be used as the basis of developing "gold standard" criteria for removing barriers to survey participation by persons with disabilities. It seems that at the national level, many countries are addressing inclusion of persons with disabilities, but more should be done. By reviewing the strategies employed by DISTAB's six national surveys, better strategies can be developed. PWD's can provide invaluable input at early stages, offer feedback in the piloting stages and suggest ways to increase response rates based on specific disabilities. Providing accessible formats is key for both the administration of the survey and in the reporting and dissemination of the survey. The analysis provided by the enhanced quality profile is useful because future surveys of disability will be informed by the innovative strategies we identified in the DISTAB surveys, and will be able to further develop their own. The five questions outlined above provide guidelines which may be the start of a "gold standard" for conducting disability surveys.

The issues for removing barriers to participation for persons with disabilities raised in the NCD report of 1998 that provide the framework used here has since been updated based on two recent international workshops on improving disability statistics and measurement, sponsored by the United Nations (UN, 2003; UN, 2004). Issues raised here provide additional recommendations for removing barriers and improving the overall quality of disability statistics. As the representativeness of PWD's improves, survey quality improves.

References

Benson, V. and Marano, M.A. Current estimates from the National Health Interview Survey, 1994. National Center for Health Statistics. Vital Health Stat 10(111). 1998.

Enquête Handicaps-Incapacités-Dépendance-Ménages, France 1999, INSEE.

Fougeryrollas, Patrick and Line Beauregard. "Disability: An Interactive Person-Environment Social Creation." *Handbook of Disability Studies*. Ed. Gary L. Albrecht, Katherine D. Seelman, and Michael Bury. Thousand Oaks: Sage, 2001. Pp. 171-194.

Greenberg, M.S. and Caroline Heick. (2002). Annual Report of the WHO Collaborating Center for the Family of International Classifications for North America, October 2001-September 2002. World Health Organization: .Geneva, Switzerland, page 15.

Hendershot, G. (1998). National Council on Disability (1998). *Reorienting disability research*. Washington DC.

Hendershot, G. (2000). National Center for Education Statistics. *Statistical Standards*. Washington DC.

NCHS. (1999a) 1995 National Health Interview Survey on Disability, Phase I and II. Reissued November, CD-ROM Series 10, No. 10B, National Center for Health Statistics, Hyattsville, MD.

NCHS (1999b). 1994 National Health Interview Survey on Disability, Phase I and II. July , CD-ROM Series 10, No. 8, National Center for Health Statistics, Hyattsville, MD.

Office of Management and Budget. (2001). "Measuring and Reporting Sources of Error in Surveys." Statistical Working Paper 31, Statistical Policy Office, Office of Information and Regulatory Affairs, July.

Schneider, M; Claassens, M.; Kimmie, Z.; Morgan, R.; Naicker, S.; Roberts, A.; McLaren P. (1999). The extent of moderate and severe reported disability and the nature of the disability experience in South Africa. CASE Report for the Department of Health, Pretoria, October, 1999.

Statistics Canada. (1991). The 1991 Health and Activity Limitation Survey (HALS), Housing, Family and Social Statistics Division, Statistics Canada.

Statistics Netherlands. (1996). Netherlands Health Interview Survey 1981 – 1995. The Hague, Sdu publishers/cbs publications 1996. ISBN 4035728122.

Swanson, G. Carrothers, L. and Mulhorn, K.A. (2002).. "Comparing Disability Survey Questions in Five Countries: A Study Using ICF to Guide Comparisons" (*The Journal of Rehabilitation Research)* Spring.

United Nations (2003). *Measurement Issues.*First Workshop for Improving Disabilty Statistics and Measurement. Bangkok, Thailand.

United Nations. (2004). *Conclusions adopted at the second workshop for improving disability statistics and measurement*. Bangkok, Thailand.

World Health Organization (WHO). (2001). *International Classification of Functioning, Disability and Health*: Geneva.

In: Towards Best Practices for Surveying People..., Volume 1 ISBN 1-60021-195-X
Editors: Thilo Kroll, David Keer et al., pp. 13-31

Chapter 2

REMOVING THE BARRIERS: MODIFYING TELEPHONE SURVEY METHODOLOGY TO INCREASE SELF-RESPONSE AMONG PEOPLE WITH DISABILITIES

Anne B. Ciemnecki and Karen A. CyBulski
Mathematica Policy Research, Inc.

ABSTRACT

Information collected directly and cost-effectively from respondents with disabilities is necessary to determine how well public programs meet their needs. Mathematica Policy Research (MPR) has been making simple modifications to survey telephone design and procedures to increase accessibility. Goals are three-fold: (1) to increase participation without using proxy respondents, (2) to keep survey costs affordable, and (3) to maintain data quality.

Minor modifications to questionnaire design to increase accessibility include short recall periods, concrete questions, elimination of high frequency sounds, inclusion of breaks to overcome fatigue, neutral encouragement, checks for unexpected responses, and structured probes. Procedural modifications include sensitivity training for interviewers, compassion fatigue support for interviewers, and modified expectations regarding time to administer questionnaires. Cooperation rates for our surveys are high (97 percent) and the vast majority of respondents answered for themselves (86 percent). Interview data are complete and accurate.

People with physical or sensory disabilities provide more complete information than those with mental illness, mental retardation or developmental disabilities, but the differences are not great. Shorter interviews (20 rather than 45 minutes) create less burden, require fewer breaks and need less interviewer encouragement. Self-respondents provide more complete information than proxy respondents.

It is both possible and desirable to collect data from large samples of people with disabilities by telephone. Respondents with disabilities do not pose extraordinary challenges for telephone surveys. The information collected from respondents with disabilities is consistent with information collected from similar populations without disabilities. Modifications to increase participation are neither costly nor difficult to implement.

Introduction

While survey research literature focuses on using surveys to identify people with disabilities and representing them statistically in population estimates (National Council on Disability 2004; National Council on Disability 1998; LaPlante and Carlson 1996; Kraus et al. 1996; Conwell Incorporated 1993; Thompson-Hoffman and Storck 1991; Zola 1990; Mathematica Policy Research 1984), the field is virtually devoid of practical recommendations for removing barriers so that people with disabilities can self-respond. The literature that is available on this topic tends to explore issues surrounding the use of assistive technology devices (most notably, TTY) and/or their potential limitations for telephone interviewing (Carlson et al. 2001; Barnett and Franks 1999; Wilson et al. 1998; Russell et al. 1997; Olsen et al. 1999; Kirchner 1998), as well as the use and selection of proxies to represent persons with disabilities in surveys (Kirchner 1998; Todorov and Kirchner 2000; Parsons et al. 2000; Black 2004).

Several other techniques used to make interviews more accessible for people with disabilities have been gleaned from the physical and cognitive challenges associated with interviewing elderly populations. For example, minimizing high-frequency sounds in surveys of elderly populations is based on information that suggests that high-frequency hearing loss is very common among adults over the age of 55 (Wingfield 1999). Moreover, interviewing elderly respondents in quiet environments is important due to "findings that speech perception in elderly adults can be especially vulnerable to the presence of background noise and speaking in a room with poor reverberation characteristics" (Wingfield 1999). In terms of questionnaire design, it has been recommended that survey researchers avoid asking questions with very long sentences, and complex syntax, to the elderly (New England States Consortium 2001; Wingfield 1999). Lastly, the use of cognitive interviewing techniques to identify comprehension problems (including screening for cognitive impairment), and "non-traditional survey approaches" (for example, allowing interviewers to rephrase a question on their own) have also been implemented in surveys of the frail elderly (New England States Consortium 2001; Ritchie 1988; Jobe et al. 1996; Jobe and Mingay 1989).

The National Institute on Disability and Rehabilitation Research (NIDRR) has recently defined a new paradigm of disability (NIDRR 2000). Under the new paradigm, disability is seen as a "deficit in the person-community relationships that should be addressed by social interactions." This represents a shift from the old paradigm that presented disability as a "deficit in an individual that prevents the individual from performing certain functions or activities." The goal of the new paradigm is to facilitate the full participation of people with disabilities. Implied by this shift are survey research methods that require new approaches to measuring disability in federally funded surveys and new approaches to making surveys accessible to people with disabilities.

In addition to the new paradigm of disability, there has been a trend toward self-directed care and self-determination, which was brought about in part by the Americans with Disabilities Act (ADA) in 1990. The law prohibits discrimination on the basis of disability in employment, state and local government, public accommodations, commercial facilities, transportation, and telecommunications. The ADA has brought with it a shift in thinking regarding the level of participation that people with disabilities have in decisions that affect their lives. Out of this shift has come the self-directed care model, which puts forth that people know their needs best and should have the right to determine the types of services that best meet these needs. Further, there has been a move toward ensuring full participation by people with disabilities in their lives. This change has brought about in an increase in the choice and control people have over meeting their support needs, increasing independence and social inclusion.

Self-directed care allows individuals to have more control over their health care decisions (CMS 2003). Programs that embrace self-directed care include the Home- and Community-Based Services (HCBS) waiver program and the Cash and Counseling demonstration. The HCBS waiver program allows individuals at risk of being placed in an institution to be cared for in their own homes, while the Cash and Counseling demonstration allows individuals to purchase supports or services that meet their personal assistance needs at home. In 2001, President Bush announced the New Freedom Initiative, which is designed to ensure that all Americans have the opportunity to learn and develop skills, engage in productive work, make choices about their daily lives, and participate fully in community life. The shift toward self-directed care and full participation by individuals with a disability further emphasizes the importance of getting survey responses directly from people with disabilities rather than from a proxy.

As part of the Centers for Medicaid and Medicare Services (CMS) evaluation of Section 1115 Medicaid Reform Demonstrations, Mathematica Policy Research, Inc. (MPR) conducted computer-assisted telephone interview (CATI) surveys with Medicaid beneficiaries in eight states.[1] Medicaid is the largest program serving the health care needs of low-income people with disabilities. People with disabilities account for approximately 15 percent of the Medicaid population (Crowley and Elias 2003). Supplemental Security Income (SSI) is a federal program funded by the Social Security Administration (SSA) that is designed to help aged, blind, and disabled people who have little or no income. SSI recipients are more likely to have diverse and complex health care needs and are frequent users of health care services (Hill and Woodridge 2000; Long et al. 2002). Their disabilities encompass physical or sensory disabilities (including blindness and deafness), mental illness, and mental retardation and other developmental disabilities (MR/DD).

In three states, Kentucky, New York, and Tennessee, separate interviews with people with disabilities were conducted to assess how SSI recipients were faring in Medicaid. To facilitate comparisons with the general Medicaid population, many of the questions that were asked of people with disabilities were identical to those asked of the general Medicaid population. Interviews with people with disabilities were not part of the original evaluation design. Therefore, the survey of the general Medicaid population was designed before the survey of people with disabilities was designed. The surveys of people with disabilities addressed access to care, quality of care, and use of health services. MPR conducted more than 4,600 interviews.

These were among the first surveys of this type to be conducted solely by telephone for people with disabilities. People with disabilities can face three broad categories of challenges

[1]This research was funded by the U.S. Department of Health and Human Services (DHHS), CMS, with additional funding from the Assistant Secretary for Planning and Evaluation (ASPE) and the Substance Abuse and Mental Health Services Administration (SAMHSA) under contract numbers 500-94-0047 and 500-95-0040. Additional funding for presentation of the findings was provided under contract number 45099-7497 by Cornell University School of Industrial and Labor Relations sponsored by the National Institute on Disability and Rehabilitation Research.

when completing an interview: communication barriers, stamina barriers, and cognitive barriers. Because of these challenges, survey researchers in the past have relied on proxy respondents or administrative data when conducting studies of this population. However, data collected through proxies or administrative records are often not of the highest quality, as research indicates that the best data are collected directly from people who are being affected by the program under study. Our goals were to (1) give respondents with disabilities the opportunity to speak for themselves regarding issues that affect their health care, and (2) provide our clients with a cost-effective way to collect data from SSI recipients. In designing our approach to the surveys, we attempted to accommodate the needs of people with disabilities by addressing the challenges that they could face when completing a telephone interview. Had these surveys been conducted face-to-face instead of by telephone, they would have cost about five to six times as much—a cost that may well have been prohibitive.

This paper discusses MPR's experience conducting telephone interviews with people with disabilities and presents recommendations for making telephone surveys more accessible. We view this as the beginning of a set of best practices for including people with disabilities in telephone surveys. We begin with a description of challenges associated with interviewing people with disabilities by telephone, describe minor modifications that can be made to instruments and procedures to remove barriers and improve self-response, and demonstrate the validity and reliability of telephone methodology for people with disabilities.

Challenges in Interviewing Disabled People by Telephone

Interviewing a population with disabilities presents several challenges. To be successful, one has to overcome challenges that may be associated with communication, stamina, or cognition.

Survey researchers collect data from persons with disabilities all the time. Usually, however, researchers are unaware that a particular respondent has a disabling condition—especially if the interview is being conducted by telephone. The problem faced in designing the SSI surveys was that *every* sample member had a disability. The specific disability and severity of disability were not available as part of the sample frame; only nominal or categorical data to describe the disability were known. Of 811 adults selected for the survey sample, 25 percent had physical or sensory disabilities, 36 percent had mental illness, 23 percent had MR/DD, and 16 percent of the adult sample had missing information on the disability condition. Moreover, there was a wide range of disabilities, with varying degrees of severity; in addition, some sample members had multiple disabling conditions. The instrumentation procedures attempted to address three broad categories of common challenges: (1) communication, (2) stamina, and (3) cognitive barriers. Communication challenges include both hearing and speech impairments. The term "stamina challenges" includes both physical and mental fatigue. Cognitive challenges include, but are not limited to, emotional disturbance, difficulty processing questions and responses, lack of complete or specific knowledge, and confusion about the purpose of the interview.

MODIFICATIONS TO INSTRUMENTATION

To overcome the challenges and to promote full participation in the study, minor modifications were made to questionnaire design and procedures to increase accessibility. The questionnaires featured four techniques designed to overcome these challenges: minimization of high-frequency sounds, interviewer checkpoints, structured probes that allowed questions to be rephrased in a standard manner, and follow-up items for non-response. In addition, questions were worded simply, clearly, briefly, and without bias, so that respondents could readily understand key terms and concepts. Questions requested information that could reasonably be expected of individuals with a disabling condition. For example, recall periods were kept short. Response categories were appropriate, mutually exclusive, and reasonably exhaustive, given the intent of the questions. Questions were accompanied by clear, concise instructions and probes so that interviewers knew exactly what was expected of them.

Minimizing High-Frequency Sounds

In the English language, consonants are more important than vowels in identifying words, and the hearing loss of high-frequency consonants (*s, z, t, f,* and *g*) is common. By replacing high frequencies with low frequencies, questions are easier to hear.[2] Following is an example of a question with numerous high-frequency sounds:

> How satisfied are you with the overall quality of care you receive as a member of *NAME OF MANAGED CARE PLAN*? Are you very satisfied, somewhat satisfied, neither satisfied nor dissatisfied, somewhat dissatisfied, or very dissatisfied?

Compare this with a version that uses low-frequency sounds:

> How would you rate the overall quality of the medical care you get as a member of *NAME OF MANAGED CARE PLAN*? Is it excellent, very good, good, fair, or poor?

While these questions are not identical, questions cannot be understood if they are not heard. Designing questions that address high-frequency hearing loss may be more important for some respondents than others. The reduction of high-frequency sounds ensures that more respondents hear the question.

Interviewer Checkpoints

Checkpoints allow interviewers to assess whether the respondent needs encouragement or is becoming too fatigued to continue the interview. The SSI surveys varied in the length of the instruments. The SSI survey in Tennessee took, on average, 44 minutes to administer; the

[2]The Canadian Task Force on Preventive Health recommends rewording sentences to avoid high-frequency sounds as a communication strategy (Patterson 1994).

SSI surveys in Kentucky and New York took 22 minutes. Pretest interviews revealed that some respondents became fatigued, especially during the longer interview. Pretesting also revealed that it was useful to provide respondents with positive feedback about completing the survey task. Comments such as, "Your answers are very helpful to this study" seemed to allay fears and put respondents at ease. Other reassuring comments that pretest interviewers used were, "There are no right or wrong answers to these questions" and "Take your time." Based on these pretest observations, three checkpoints were included in the interviews. The checkpoints ensured that interviewers stop and assess the respondent's ability to continue. They also provided prompts for interviewers to provide encouragement when necessary. Interviewers were required to record their actions at each checkpoint: Interviewer Checkpoint: Does The Respondent Seem Fatigued, Confused, Or Need Encouragement?

Fatigue Probe

1) Are you feeling tired, or can we continue?
2) Would you like to take a break? I can hold on.
3) Would you like to continue the interview another time?

Encouragement Probe

1) Your answers are very helpful for this study.
2) There are no right or wrong answers to these questions.

Interviewer Action

Not Fatigued, No Encouragement Provided	00
Fatigued And Wants To Be Called Back	01
Fatigued But Can Continue	02
Gave Encouragement	03

Despite their disabling conditions, about three-quarters of the respondents were able to complete the 22-minute interview without special intervention from the interviewer (Table 1).

About half of the respondents completed the 44-minute interview without needing special intervention. These differences persisted across all disabling conditions.

Table 1. Interviewer Actions At Checkpoints

	Total		Physical/Sensory		Mental Illness		Schizophrenia		MR/DD[a]		Unknown	
	22 Min	44 Min	22 Min	44 Min	22 Min	44 Min	22 Min	44 Min	22 Min	44 Min	22 Min	44 Min
Total Respondents (N =)	2,852	916	795	282	842	288	321	NA	510	235	384	111
Percent Who Needed:												
No Iintervention	73%	51%	70%	50%	69%	54%	91%	NA	72%	49%	72%	52%
Some Intervention	28%	49%	30%	50%	31%	46%	9%	NA	27%	51%	27%	48%
Encouragement only	27%	38%	29%	38%	31%	34%	9%	NA	27%	42%	27%	35%
Callbacks	0%	11%	0%	12%	0%	11%	0%	NA	0%	9%	0%	13%
No intervention but showed fatigue	1%	0%	1%	0%	0%	1%	0%	NA	0%	0%	0%	0%

[a]Mental retardation and other developmental disabilities.

Not one respondent needed a break during the 22-minute interview (Table 2). Eleven percent of the respondents needed a break during the longer interview. Of these respondents, a second break was needed by more than half because their stamina was too little or attention span was too short to complete the interview in one session. Almost one-fourth of those who needed one break, however, were able to continue without further intervention. All respondents who needed a break completed the interview on a subsequent call. While the percentage who needed a break did not vary much by disabling condition, respondents with physical or sensory disabilities were most likely to need more than one break. These respondents tended to tire quickly or have difficulty using the phone for prolonged periods. Respondents with severe and persistent mental illness were most able to continue with no further intervention after a break.

Interviewers provided encouragement about one-third less often during the shorter interview than during the longer for those with physical or sensory disabilities or MR/DD. Respondents with mental illness needed almost as much encouragement during the shorter interview as during the longer one. This may be because the shorter interview focused on issues of mental and behavioral health. A subsample of respondents with schizophrenia needed almost no support or intervention during the 22-minute interview. Eighty-two percent of the schizophrenic subgroup reported taking a medication for a mental or emotional health problem. This medication may have had enough of a positive impact to enable the group to complete the interview easily, even though other analysis suggests that this group was not receiving adequate care for their illness (Mitchell et al. 2003). There was no 44-minute interview for this subgroup.

Table 2.Outcomes For Sample Members Who Needed Callbacks (In The 44-Minute Interview)

	Total	Physical/ Sensory	Mental Illness	MR/DD[a]	Unknown
Respondents Who Needed Callbacks (N =)	100%	34%	32%	20%	14%
Of those who needed callbacks, percent who:					
Needed a second callback	56%	62%	44%	55%	71%
Continued with no further intervention	23%	12%	34%	25%	21%
Continued with only encouragement	21%	26%	22%	20%	7%

Generally, the interviewers perceived that respondents were happy to be interviewed and were reluctant to stop. Even though respondents to the shorter interview did not need breaks, we recommend including the checkpoints in surveys of people with disabilities. Interviewers also reported that the checkpoints caused them to slow down the pace of the interview while also serving as a reminder that they were speaking with respondents who were likely to experience difficulties. Interviewers reported that the encouragement was especially helpful for respondents who did not know the answer to a question or series of questions. For these respondents, interviewers discovered that the following sentence helped respondents relax and continue: "I know these questions are hard to answer, and you are doing your best." The interviewers strongly recommended the use of encouragement in future surveys of populations with disabilities.

Structured Probes

A series of structured probes was used to keep the interview for the respondents with disabilities as comparable as possible to the interview administered to the general population of Medicaid recipients. The majority of questions worked well for most of the respondents with disabilities. Nevertheless, some respondents needed to have concepts defined. To the extent possible, the wording of the original question was preserved and supplemented with standardized definitions and probes that would clarify key concepts. To ensure that interviewers used them consistently, the probes appeared on the CATI screens in the order that interviewers should use them. If none of the probes helped the respondent, the interviewer was allowed to rephrase the question in a way she thought the respondent would understand. In the following examples, the new, structured probes appear in boldface:

Example 1

For How Many Of The Last Twelve Months—That Is, Since Month And Year 12 Months Ago—Have You Been Enrolled In Name Of Behavioral Health Plan?

PROBE: For Which Months Have You Been Enrolled?
Probe: For How Long Have You Been Enrolled? Have You Been Enrolled In Name Of Behavioral Health Plan All Of That Time?

Example 2

During the last twelve months, was there any time when you took less than the recommended dosage or took a prescription medication less frequently than recommended, so the medication would last longer?

PROBE: Stretched the medication so it would last longer?

Examples 3-5

Because of a physical, mental, or emotional problem, do you currently get help or supervision from another person

managing money?
PROBE: Counting money, getting the correct change, or paying bills?
using the telephone?
PROBE: Answering the phone or dialing numbers?

doing heavy housework?
PROBE: Like scrubbing floors or washing windows?

Example 6

How long ago did you have your blood pressure taken by a doctor or other health professional?

PROBE: When was the last time you had your blood pressure taken?
PROBE: The doctor or nurse puts a cuff around your arm, pumps it up, and listens with a stethoscope?

Interviewers reported that they always read the main question first but often read the probe before waiting for the respondent to answer the main question, because, after establishing rapport with the respondent, they determined that the respondent needed the clarifying probes. Interviewers reported that the structured probes were usually sufficient for people with disabilities, and that they rephrased questions most often for a subpopulation of Russian respondents in New York City and Westchester County. The rephrasing was due to language barriers, not disabilities. Interviewers were not required to record how they rephrased questions.

Follow-Up Items for Non-Response

While item non-response was low (less than 3 percent for most items), some respondents, especially those who lacked complete and specific knowledge, had difficulty providing precise responses to questions about income, length of time spent waiting at the doctor's office, or out-of-pocket medical expenses. To minimize item non-response, follow-up questions were added to the survey instrument for continuous variables. If a respondent could not provide an exact amount, the "Don't know" response was followed with a modified version of the question that offered response categories. The upper and lower bounds of each category were based on the ranges the analysts used. The follow-up questions resolved about three-quarters of item non-response.

Modifications to Procedures

In addition to modifying instrumentation, survey staffing and procedures were modified to ensure high-quality data. Special interviewer training, relaxed interviewer productivity standards, continuity of contacts, and an easy-to-understand advance letter all contributed to respondent and interviewer comfort with the data collection.

Interviewer Selection, Training, and Supervision

The SSI surveys were staffed with experienced interviewers, but they had not had special training in working with people with disabilities. The training program consisted of giving the usual background and purpose of the study, a question-by-question review of the instrument, contact protocols, refusal avoidance, and practice interviews. In addition, trainers addressed challenges the interviewers were likely to face. Training began with a sensitivity exercise designed to demonstrate that interviewers should be kind and have unconditional positive regard for respondents regardless of their limitations. Trainers stressed that the biggest barriers people with disabilities face and the hardest barriers to remove are others' negative attitudes and erroneous images of them. Interviewers were trained to use positive rather than patronizing language and were encouraged to place their focus on the individual first and the disability last.

Trainers presented the three general challenges that persons with disabilities face completing telephone interviews and provided guidance for overcoming each one. Communication challenges were divided into hearing and speech impairments. To overcome hearing impairments, interviewers learned (1) to use a normal tone of voice and not restrict conversations to single-syllable words, (2) to use controls on headsets to amplify outgoing sounds, and (3) to use a text telephone (TTY/TTD) relay operator, if necessary. To overcome speech impairments, interviewers learned (1) to use controls on the headsets to amplify incoming sounds; (2) to not be afraid to ask the respondent to repeat what he or she said; (3) to be patient, because speech patterns become easier to discern after a few minutes; (4) to repeat aloud what they did hear and understand if clarification is needed; and (5) to not pretend to understand something they did not. Instead, they were to go back and build from the point at which they did understand. Trainers demonstrated that people with speech impairments may be unable to monitor their tone of voice. For example, a person with cerebral palsy may seem angry, when actually she or he is not, and people who slur words may seem drunk when they are not. Interviewers were encouraged not to make assumptions about people based on their tone of voice. This part of the training was reinforced by having interviewers monitor an interview with a respondent with a severe speech impairment.

To overcome stamina challenges, interviewers were trained to be aware of behaviors that might suggest the respondent was too fatigued to continue. For instance, agitation and distraction can signal that the respondent is ready for a break. Interviewers were encouraged to ask whether the respondent needed to schedule another time to continue, and to set appointments for times when the respondent was most alert.

To overcome cognitive challenges, the training focused on nonbiased, nondirective probing methods (silence, repeating the question, repeating the response categories, asking for more information, stressing generality, stressing subjectivity, and zeroing in) and using active listening skills and patience. The trainers showed interviewers (1) how to keep the respondent free of distractions, (2) instructed them to say the respondent's name often, and (3) suggested that they not exaggerate the inflection or tone of their voice (such exaggerations call attention to themselves and can be distracting and confusing). When the survey was over, interviewers reported that interviewing was not as difficult as the training suggested.

Production Standards

Conducting telephone interviews with people with disabilities can be challenging even for experienced, well-trained interviewers. Interviews take longer because questions need to be repeated, and multiple sessions may be required. The estimates of respondent burden submitted to OMB reflected the extra time needed. Extra efforts were made to support the interviewers and reduce stress and burnout. To accomplish this, the usual performance measures (such as hours per completed interview) were eased. Supervisors reminded interviewers that break-offs were acceptable and desirable if respondents were fatigued. Supervisors and colleagues provided support during and after interviews and at regular debriefing sessions.

Contact Procedures

In an effort to increase respondent trust and rapport, the standard contact procedures were modified for this study. Typically, if a callback is required in order to continue the interview or reach the respondent at a better time, it is as likely as not that a different interviewer will make the follow-up phone call. For this study, once contact was made with a respondent, that case was assigned to the interviewer who made contact. Every effort was made to maintain the interviewer continuity.

An advance letter was sent to all beneficiaries in the survey sample prior to the interview. The advance letter explained the purpose of the survey, offered assurances of confidentiality, and included a toll-free number for respondents to call with questions or to complete the interview at their convenience. Sending a letter in advance of the telephone contact also serves to increase the legitimacy of the survey.

A proxy respondent is a person who completes an interview on behalf of a sample member. Proxy respondents were recruited when interviewers learned that sample members were unable to complete the interview themselves due to a physical or mental condition such as hearing impairment or dementia. Eligible proxies included individuals familiar with the health care experiences of the sample member. They were often the spouses, children, or other relatives and friends of the sample member. Overall, 17 percent of the interviews were completed by proxy respondents.

Interviewer Assessments

Interviewers were asked to rate the respondents' ability to understand and answer questions. They rated both self-respondents and proxies. Interviewers rated the vast majority of self-respondents (80 percent) as Good to Excellent (Table 3). It is not surprising that those with physical or sensory disabilities earned the highest ratings of the three groups—88 percent were rated Good to Excellent. Even among self-respondents with MR/DD, the group with the lowest percentage of Good to Excellent ratings, almost three-quarters (74 percent) were rated as Good to Excellent respondents. Self-respondents with MR/DD were, however, less likely to get Excellent ratings than the other two groups. Twenty-two percent earned Excellent ratings, compared to 33 percent of those with mental illness and 39 percent of those with physical or sensory disabilities. Proxy respondents were only slightly more likely than self-respondents to earn Good to Excellent ratings (85 percent versus 80 percent) but were much more likely to earn Excellent ratings (48 versus 32 percent). Only 5 percent of self-respondents and 4 percent of proxies were considered poor respondents. These assessments reinforce that seeking self-response is desirable.

Table 3. Interviewer Assessment of Respondent's Ability to Understand and Answer Questions

	Total	Excellent	Very Good	Good	Fair	Poor
Self-Respondents						
All	919	32%	25%	23%	14%	5%
Physical	283	39%	30%	19%	9%	3%
Mental illness	288	33%	23%	23%	16%	5%
MR/DD	237	22%	26%	26%	18%	8%
Unknown	111	32%	19%	27%	15%	7%
Proxy Respondents						
All	151	48%	21%	16%	11%	4%
Physical	22	68%	9%	14%	5%	5%
Mental illness	34	41%	24%	18%	15%	3%
MR/DD	78	45%	23%	17%	12%	4%
Unknown	17	47%	24%	12%	12%	6%

MEASURES OF DATA QUALITY

Data quality can be measured in terms of high response rates, both to the survey (unit response) and to specific survey questions (item response), and in terms of the reliability and validity of the data. The data collected by telephone from people with disabilities met the same unit and item response rate, reliability, and validity standards that you would expect of the general population.

Self-Response

Respondents appreciated the opportunity to participate in these surveys. Table 4 shows response rates, cooperation rates, and self-response rates by state, as well as the type of disability, as defined in the SSI files.[1] The cooperation rates were, on average, 95 percent, ranging from 94 percent for respondents with mental illness, to 97 percent for respondents

[1] MPR strictly adheres to AAPOR's standard definitions of outcome rates for surveys (AAPOR 2004). Response rates are defined as completed interviews divided by the number of interviews completed plus the number of non-interviews plus all cases of unknown eligibility. The cooperation rate is the number of completed interviews divided by all eligible cases ever contacted. The self-response rate is the number of sample members who responded for themselves divided by the number of completed interviews.

with MR/DD. The average self-response rate, though 83 percent, varied considerably by type of disabling condition. Those with physical or sensory disabilities were the most likely to self-respond (90 percent); 87 percent of those with mental illness self-responded; and 73 percent of those with MR/DD answered for themselves. The only notable source of non-response was the inability to locate sample members by telephone. Those with physical or sensory disabilities were the most likely to be located (73 percent), while only 67 percent of those with mental illness or MR/DD could be located. Sample frames were state Medicaid administrative records. Although the data quality varied from state to state, in all three states the files had cases that either lacked addresses or telephone numbers, or they contained inaccurate contact information.

Table 4.Response Rates, Cooperation Rates, and Self-Response Rates, by State and Type of Disability

	Response Rate	Cooperation Rate	Self-Response Rate
Tennessee	67.3%	96.5%	87.0%
Physical/sensory	70.2%	95.3%	93.4%
Mental illness	67.5%	96.2%	90.4%
MR/DD[a]	62.0%	97.8%	81.4%
Unknown	70.3%	96.9%	80.7%
Kentucky	74.3%	97.4%	83.9%
Physical/sensory	84.4%	98.5%	92.7%
Mental illness	71.9%	97.3%	85.8%
MR/DD	72.2%	96.5%	75.8%
Unknown	71.5%	97.5%	74.6%
New York City	57.5%	92.8%	78.8%
Physical/sensory	60.9%	91.8%	86.9%
Mental illness	53.3%	87.4%	85.1%
MR/DD	55.9%	97.3%	69.0%
Unknown	62.1%	94.9%	75.4%
Westchester County	59.0%	92.5%	80.7%
Physical/sensory	61.4%	93.1%	86.9%
Mental illness	56.0%	90.8%	87.9%
MR/DD	64.9%	96.3%	56.1%
Unknown	56.4%	91.5%	76.7%
Total	65.7%	95.3%	83.0%
Physical/sensory	69.6%	95.1%	90.4%
Mental illness	64.5%	94.3%	87.0%
MR/DD	64.0%	97.0%	72.7%
Unknown	65.3%	95.4%	77.1%

Both the response and cooperation rates for the surveys of people with disabilities were higher than those for surveys of the general Medicaid population that used the same sample frame.

In Tennessee, for example, the response rate for the survey of the general Medicaid population conducted one year earlier was 57.4 percent (versus 67.3 percent), while the cooperation rate was 87.7 percent (versus 96.5 percent). The locatability rates were identical. Given that the cooperation rates were uniformly high, response rates for both surveys would have been higher if the contact data on the state administrative files were accurate (CyBulski et al. 2001). CMS currently has an interagency agreement with the Social Security Administration to obtain contact data from their files. These agreements were not in place when these surveys were conducted.

Item Non-Response

To determine whether specific types of questions were especially difficult to answer by phone and, if so, for whom they were difficult, item non-response was examined. Overall, item non-response was less than 3 percent. Response rates to items (i.e., answered something other than "do not know" or "refused") were examined by topical areas of the survey. Topical areas included access, attitudes, choice, specialists, satisfaction, demographics, mental health care, quality of care, paying for care, and health and functioning. Respondents were best able to answer questions about payment for care, demographics, and health and functioning. For these items, more than 96 percent of the self-respondents answered 95 percent or more of the items on their individual interviews. Both demographics and health and functioning are salient, easy-to-answer items. Most respondents did not have out-of-pocket costs to report and skipped most of these items.

The items next easiest to answer concerned attitudes, mental health care, and quality of care. At least 87 percent of the self-respondents answered 95 percent or more of the items in these topic areas. The most difficult questions to answer were those about choice of a managed care organization and primary care physician. Only half of the respondents were able to answer 95 percent or more of the items in this area. This is likely because the questions implicitly have a long recall period and because some respondents may have had others help them make those choices. For all but one topic area—use of specialists—the item non-response rate was higher for proxies than for self-respondents. Proxies lacked information about choice, demographics, and mental health care. Generally, respondents with physical and sensory disabilities had higher item response rates than respondents with mental illness and MR/DD. Self-respondents with mental illness had a particularly hard time with quantitative questions—33 percent could not answer at least 95 percent of the items on their individual interviews.

As a benchmark, item response rates for self-responding adults were compared to item response rates for parents of disabled children.[2] Because parents are involved in their children's care, we would expect them to be able to answer all these questions without difficulty. Proxies for children have slightly higher item response rates than adult self-respondents in half of the topic areas and are much better able to answer items with long recall periods, questions that require quantitative responses, and questions about specialty care.

This information suggests that most people with disabilities can answer most questions about most topics. But, minimizing proxy use, asking about easy, salient concepts, and keeping the recall period short are important ways to minimize non-response in surveys of people with disabilities.

Next, patterns of answers across pairs of questions were compared for consistency. Responses were found to be consistent at an aggregate level. Specifically, there was consistency between reported factual measures of access to care and satisfaction with access to care. These comparisons are qualitative, rather than relying on statistical tests. Respondents who rated travel time to providers as fair or poor also reported having longer travel times to

[2]Disabled children were also included in these surveys. Parents always served as proxies for their children. These analyses refer to the adult sample only. Except for this reference, proxy use in this paper refers to proxies who responded on behalf of adults who could not respond for themselves.

providers, on average. Respondents who rated time spent waiting in the doctor's office as fair or poor also reported having longer waiting times, on average. Respondents who rated access to specialist care as fair or poor also reported that their managed care plan failed to refer them to a specialist, referred them to the wrong type of specialist, or delayed approval for specialist care. Those who chose their mental health provider tended to rate more highly the choice of mental providers, relative to those who were assigned to providers.

CONCLUSION

It is in our best interest as survey researchers to make surveys accessible to a broad spectrum of respondents at the lowest cost possible. Furthermore, it is our responsibility to collect the highest-quality data possible. Most of the time, data of the highest quality can be collected directly from the people who are affected by the programs we study. We have demonstrated that, through careful instrument design and survey procedures, it is possible to conduct telephone interviews with people with disabilities. Shorter interviews cause less respondent burden and can be conducted with fewer break-offs and less need for encouragement from the interviewer than longer interviews.

Our experience suggests that states can use telephone surveys to assess the performance of people with disabilities in federally sponsored health programs. It was feasible to interview large samples of disabled beneficiaries over the telephone. Furthermore, this interview mode provided information that appears to be as analytically useful as the information collected using telephone surveys of the general Medicaid population or using in-person interviews with people with disabilities.

In the end, the data proved sufficient for evaluating how the SSI population is faring in the Medicaid programs. The data permitted an analysis of the diverse needs of disabled SSI beneficiaries, their participation in selecting their health plans and providers, and their access to care. The data also indicated that access to care and satisfaction levels differed among the beneficiaries in different managed care plans. Thus, the data collected through the telephone survey met the ultimate test in terms of providing useful information for assessing and planning managed care (Hill et al. 2000; Draper et al. 2001; Long et al. 2002; Mitchell et al. 2003; Bir et al. 2004).

The major challenges in using telephone interviews to collect information from people with disabilities are the same as in general surveys. In particular, poor contact information in the state administrative files was largely responsible for limiting the overall response rate. Other challenges that are typical of Medicaid-related surveys, not just those of people with disabilities, included questions with long recall periods, such as those required to assess plan choice at the time a beneficiary enrolled, quantitative questions, such as the number of physician office visits or out-of-pocket expenditures during the last six months, and measures of satisfaction with complex phenomena, such as experiences with an insurer or health care provider. The disabled beneficiaries themselves do not appear to pose an extraordinary challenge to a telephone survey. The high cooperation rate of 97 percent for the SSI population exceeded the rate for Tennessee's general Medicaid population, and the vast majority, 83 percent, responded for themselves.

Despite the many challenges stemming from the general nature of this survey, the telephone interviews appear to have produced data that are relatively complete and accurate. People with disabilities that arose primarily from physical and sensory conditions tended to provide more complete information than those with mental illness or MR/DD, although the differences were not great.

In reviewing the implementation and results of the survey, we feel that its success lies in several basic operational features. First, the design focused on concrete questions and kept the short recall periods used in surveys of the general Medicaid population. Second, interviewer training focused not only on the actual questions in the questionnaire, but also on strategies for dealing with the challenges encountered while interviewing people with disabilities. Finally, the actual implementation included respondent breaks and other features that helped people with limited stamina or cognitive difficulties to complete long interviews.

Many of these interviewing accommodations are useful not only for people with disabilities, but for the general population as well, and could be best viewed as universal design. The concept of universal design allows a product or environment to be usable by as many people as possible regardless of age, ability, or situation (Universal Design Education Online 2005). This universal design would make it easier for people with disabilities to participate in general population surveys and would also improve interviews for all participants.

As successful as these first attempts to interview people with disabilities solely by telephone were, we recognize that not all people with disabilities can complete a telephone interview. We strongly advocate self-response rather than proxy response and suggest several modifications to the telephone-only technique to accomplish this in future surveys. First, allow for "assisted" interviews. These are different from proxy interviews because sample members are present when the questions are asked, and they try to respond for themselves. The assistant, typically a family member, provides encouragement, interpretation, and verification of answers if needed. Second, combine proxy and self-response by telephone. Even when a proxy must be used for most of the interview, the sample member can be given the opportunity to answer items on satisfaction with services, decisions he or she made, and other attitudinal or sensitive items. Finally, mixed-mode designs add in-person or self-administered (paper or web-based) interviews for individuals who cannot respond via telephone.

ACKNOWLEDGEMENTS

Many people contributed to the success of these surveys and helped make this report possible. First and foremost, the authors would like to thank the individuals who participated in the interviews and shared a part of their lives with us. We especially thank the interviewers and locators, Debbie Reese of Mathematica Policy Research, Inc. (MPR) and Richard Heman-Ackah, formerly at MPR, who led the data collection effort, and Stephanie Naber, formerly at MPR, who led the locating effort. Our colleagues at MPR, Judith Wooldridge, Craig Thornton, Barbara Kolln, and Walter Williams; Steven Hill, of the Agency for Health Research and Quality and Michael Sinclair, of the Department of Labor, both formerly at MPR; Teresa Coughlin and Sharon Long of the Urban Institute; and Jan Mitchell of RTI

International all played key roles in the project and provided valuable insight. Rita Stapulonis and Ethan Ellis made valuable suggestions on how to improve this report. Dawn Smith worked on document preparation. We appreciate the support of our project officers, Paul Boben and Penny Pine, at the Centers for Medicare and Medicaid Services.

REFERENCES

American Association for Public Opinion Research. "Standard Definitions: Final Dispositions of Cases Codes and Outcome Rates for Surveys." Lenexa, KS: American Association for Public Opinion Research, 2004.

Bir A., S. Hoover, and J.B. Mitchell. "Four-State Comparison of Access, Utilization and Quality of Care for Adults and Children with SSI." Final report. Waltham, MA: RTI International, July 2004.

Barnett, S., and Franks, P. Telephone Ownership and Deaf People: Implications for Telephone Surveys. *American Journal of Public Health 89*(11), 1999, pp. 1754-1756.

Black, Ken. "Measurement Issues". Presented at the First Workshop for Improving Disability Statistics and Measurement. Bangkok, May 24-28, 2004.

Carlson, Dawn, Nathaniel Ehrlich, Betty Jo Berland, and Nell Bailey. "Assistive Technology Survey Results: Continued Benefits and Needs Reported by Americans With Disabilities". September 27, 2001.

Centers for Medicare & Medicaid Services, Division of Disabled and Elderly Health Programs. "Home and Community-Based Services: From Institutional Care to Self-Directed Supports and Services.May 2003.

Conwell Incorporated. Disability Statistics. *Brief, XIV*, Number 8. Washington, D.C.: National Institute on Disability and Rehabilitation Research, 1993.

Crowley, Jeffrey S., and Risa Elias. "Medicaid's Role for People with Disabilities. The Kaiser Commission on Medicaid and the Uninsured, August 2003.

Draper, Debra, Karen A. CyBulski, and Anne Ciemnecki. "How Are People with Mental Illness Faring in TennCare?" Princeton, NJ: Mathematica Policy Research, Inc., April 2001.

Hill, Steven, Judith Wooldridge, Anne Ciemnecki, Karen A. CyBulski, Barbara Kolln, Michael Sinclair, and Craig Thornton. "SSI Enrollees in TennCare: Room for Improvement." Princeton, NJ: Mathematica Policy Research, Inc., March 2000.

Jobe, J., and Mingay, D.J. Cognitive Techniques in Interviewing Older People, In N. Schwartz and S. Sudman (Eds.), *Answering Questions: Methodology for Determining Cognitive and Communicative Process in Survey Research.* 1989, pp. 197-219, San Francisco: Jossey-Bass Publishers.

Jobe, J., and Mingay, D. Cognitive Laboratory Approach to Designing Questionnaires for Surveys of the Elderly. *Public Health Reports 105*(5), 1990, pp. 518-523.

Kirchner, C. Improving Research by Assuring Access. *Footnotes* 26(7), 7, 1998.

Kraus, Lewis, E., Susan Stoddard, Ph.D., and David Gilmartin. "Chartbook on Disability in the United States, 1996". National Institute on Disability and Rehabilitation Research. Washington, D.C.: 1996.

LaPlante, M., and Carlson, D. Disability in the United States: Prevalence and Causes, 1992. *Disability Statistics Report (7)*. Washington, D.C.: U.S. Department of Education, National Institute on Disability and Rehabilitation Research, 1996.

Long, Sharon K., Teresa A. Coughlin, and Stephanie J. Kendall. "Access to Care Among Disabled Adults on Medicaid." *Health Care Financing Review, 23*(2), pp.159-173, 2002.

Mathematica Policy Research, Inc. Digest of Data on Persons With Disabilities. Washington, D.C.: June 1984.

Mitchell, J.B., S. Hoover, and A. Bir. "Poor and Disabled in Rural Kentucky: Access to Care for SSI Adults and Children." Waltham, MA: RTI International, January 2003.

National Council on Disability. Reorienting Disability Research. Washington, D.C.: April 1, 1998.

National Council on Disability. Improving Federal Disability Data. Washington, D.C.: Jaunary 9, 2004.

New England States Consortium. "Designing Effective Survey Methods for Frail Elders". *Symposium Proceedings*. August 2001.

Olsen, L., et al. The National Immunization Survey: Development of Strategies to Include Deaf Respondents in an RDD Telephone Survey. Presented at the American Public Health Association Conference, Chicago, 1999.

Parsons, Jennifer A., Sara Baum, and Timothy P. Johnson. "Inclusion of Disabled Populations in Social Surveys: Review and Recommendations". Survey Research Laboratory, University of Illinois at Chicago, December 2000.

Patterson, C. "Prevention of Hearing Impairment and Disability in the Elderly. In *Canadian Guide to Clinical Preventive Health Care,* Canadian Task Force on the Periodic Health Examination. Ottawa: *Health Canada*, 1994, pp. 954-963.

Ritchie, K. The Screening of Cognitive Impairment in the Elderly: A Critical Review of Current Methods. *Journal of Clinical Epidemiology*, *41*, pp. 635-643.

Russell, N., Hendershot, G.E., LeClere, F., Howie, J., and Adler, M. Trends and Differential Use of Assistive Technology Devices: United States, 1994. *Advance Data from Vital and Health Statistics, No. 292*. Hyattsville, MD: National Center for Health Statistics, 1997.

Thompson-Hoffman, S., Storck, I.F., (Eds). *Disability in the United States: A Portrait from National Data.* New York: Springer Publishing Company, 1991.

Todorov, A., and Kirchner, C. Bias in Proxies' Reports of Disability: Data from the National Health Interview Survey on Disability. *American Journal of Public Health 90*, pp. 1248-1253, 2000.

Universal Design Education Online. www.udeducation.org/ Accessed on September 6, 2005.

U.S. Department of Education, Office of Special Education and Rehabilitative Services, National Institute on Disability and Rehabilitation Research. *Long-Range Plan, 1999-2003.* Washington, DC: U.S. Government Printing Office, 2000.

Wilson, Barbara Foley, Senda Benaissa, Karen Whitaker, Paul Beatty, and Gerry Hendershot. "Improving the Feasibility of Including Deaf Respondents in Telephone Surveys". Paper presented at 53rd Annual Conference of the American Association of Public Opinion Research, 1998.

Wingfield, Arthur. "Comprehending Spoken Questions: Effects of Cognitive and Sensory Change in Adult Aging". *Cognition, Aging, and Self-Reports,* edited by Norbert Schwarz, Denise Park, Barbel Knauper, and Seymour Sudman. Psychology Press, A Member of the Taylor and Francis Group 1999.

In: Towards Best Practices for Surveying People..., Volume 1 ISBN 1-60021-195-X
Editors: Thilo Kroll, David Keer et al., pp. 33-45

Chapter 3

CHALLENGES IN DEFINING RESPONDENT POPULATIONS IN A WEB SURVEY OF INDIVIDUALS WITH PSYCHIATRIC DISABILITIES*

Judith A. Cook[1], Dennis D. Grey[1], Genevieve Fitzgibbon[1], Drew Batteiger[1], Sylvia Caras[1], Howard Dansky[2] and Frances Priester[3]

[1] University of Illinois at Chicago
[2] Services, Technical Assistance and Resources for Human Development
[3] Washington, DC Department of Mental Health, Office of Consumer and Family Affairs

ABSTRACT

Web-based surveys may offer advantages in recruiting respondents and administering questionnaires for some populations whose disabilities are hidden or stigmatized. This study used Web-based survey technology to study self-determination among individuals with psychiatric disabilities. The web-based survey approach proved to be successful in recruiting a large number of study participants in a cost-effective manner. The mode of survey presentation allowed administration of a protocol with complex skip patterns yet accompanied by very little respondent burden. However, we also noted some concerns with regard to the overrepresentation in this study of college-educated women from Caucasian background. Another concern was the fairly high level of self-determination reported by the study respondents while a large volume of literature is pointing to the low levels of self-determination among individuals with psychiatric disabilities. Perhaps self-determination is higher among Internet users, or among some sub-groups of individuals with severe mental illnesses. While it may be fruitful to explore the use of Web-based surveys with psychiatric populations, caution must be applied by researchers in the interpretation of findings if respondents with different self-

* Funded by Cooperative Agreement # H133B000700 from the National Institute on Disability and Rehabilitation Research, U.S. Department of Education, and the Center for Mental Health Services, Substance Abuse and Mental Health Services Administration. The contents of this paper are solely the responsibility of the authors and do not necessarily represent the official views of any federal agency.

identifications have different background characteristics and clinical experiences and, most importantly, different levels of self-determination.

INTRODUCTION

Efforts over the past several decades to increase integration of individuals with disabilities into the political, economic, and social arenas of American society have raised concerns about self-determination. Self-determination refers to a person's ability to freely make important life choices such as where to live, with whom to associate, what kind of work to do, and whether to receive disability-related services. Given the difficulty of researching some populations whose disabilities are hidden or stigmatized, a Web-based survey approach may offer advantages in recruiting respondents and administering the research protocol. This study used Web-based survey technology to study self-determination among individuals with psychiatric disabilities. The study's methodological approach provided an opportunity to identify some of the advantages as well as the pitfalls of surveying people with psychiatric disabilities using Web recruitment and survey methodology.

REVIEW OF THE LITERATURE

Self-determination involves having the resources to create a good life, make responsible decisions, and choose whether and how one receives services and support for mental health problems (Rothman et al., 1996). It encompasses concepts that are central to existence in a democratic society, including freedom of choice, civil rights, independence, and self-direction (Tower, 1994). In the United States today however, low levels of self-determination among people with psychiatric disabilities have been well documented (Cook and Jonikas, 2002). Many individuals with this disability live in conditions of poverty and cope with a host of unmet needs (Ware and Goldfinger, 1997). This significantly hinders their ability to have maximal independence and to make meaningful decisions regarding their own lives (del Vecchio, Fricks et al., 2000). They experience higher than average levels of unemployment, incarceration, chronic medical illness, and social isolation (United States Department of Education, 2000). Perceptions persist that, compared to other groups, they are not as deserving of housing assistance and support (Center for Mental Health Services, 1998), so that sizable numbers are homeless or live in unstable housing (Rosenfield, 1991) while others are forced to reside with parents well into adulthood (Cook, Hoffschmidt et al., 1992).

Given the disadvantaged position of individuals with psychiatric disabilities in American society, recruiting them for research studies can be especially difficult. Because of the highly stigmatized nature of mental illness, individuals are often reluctant to self-identify as having a major mental disorder. Yet, since mental illness is a "hidden" disability, such self-identification is critical to researchers who are seeking to study this population. Another concern in research regarding this group is protection of confidentiality given the negative reactions of others to being publicly identified as having mental health problems. An additional barrier is that, even after agreeing to participate in research, subjects may feel constrained by positive response bias to report socially desirable attitudes and behaviors, further distorting study results.

Many of these problems can be addressed by employing Internet survey methodology in which potential respondents are recruited online and complete the survey instrument via Web technology. This methodological approach can be superior to others for several reasons. First, the Internet has been shown to be useful for studying specialized, difficult-to-reach populations (Kraut, Banaji, Bruckman et al., 2004) such as members of socially stigmatized communities who might hesitate to self-identify and permit face-to-face contact with researchers (Murray and Fisher, 2002; Subramanian et al., 1997). In one study, researchers soliciting a gay and lesbian sample for a study of sexual behavior were successful in using a Web-based approach to collect one of the largest such samples to date (Epstein and Klinkenberg, 2002). Second, use of the Internet to collect data affords research participants a degree of anonymity and confidentiality that exceeds many other approaches such as face-to-face interviews or even mail surveys (Fawcett and Buhle, 1995). For example, in one Internet survey of oncology nursing experts (Im and Chee, 2002) the investigators reported that ensuring confidentiality was relatively simple as long as data collection consisted entirely of anonymous communication during completing and submission of survey responses. Third, research via the Internet is associated with less social pressure due to lack of interaction with and distance from the researcher (Kraut et al., 2004). In comparing responses of research participants to paper and pencil versus Web-based surveys, Joinson (1999) found that respondents reported lower social desirability and social anxiety when data were gathered via the Internet. These advantages, however, must be weighed against disadvantages of web-based surveys including problems of self-selection leading to sample and response biases (Gonzalez, 2002), inability to monitor drop-outs (Birnbaum, 2004), low response rates (Ranchhod and Zhou, 2001), lack of control over the data collection setting (Kraut et al., 2004), and difficulties in protection of human subjects (Im and Chee, 2004).

The primary purpose of the present analysis was to assess the utility of studying individuals with psychiatric disabilities using a Web-based approach. Three basic questions were addressed. First, would Web survey technology reach individuals with psychiatric disabilities and would they agree to participate? Second, how would individuals self-identify themselves in relation to their mental health problems? Third, would those with different self-identifications differ from each other demographically, clinically, and in their level of self-determination? The following section describes the procedures used to address these research questions.

METHODOLOGY

Sampling Strategy

A convenience sample of individuals with psychiatric disabilities was obtained through announcements posted to a number of mental health listservs and websites, sent to members of the University of Illinois at Chicago National Research and Training Center on Psychiatric Disability (UIC NRTC) mailing list, and advertised in newsletters targeted to people with psychiatric disabilities and other mental health stakeholders. This announcement explained the purpose of the survey, described eligible respondents, and directed interested participants to a secure Web address where they could complete the survey online with full anonymity. Potential respondents with questions or those having difficulty completing the survey were provided with contact information for UIC NRTC staff.

Web Survey Procedures

The survey website could be visited by anyone with access to the Internet. At the website, participants were presented with instructions and an explanation of the purpose of the study, followed by a series of survey questions that took approximately ten to twenty minutes to complete, depending on the "skip pattern" created by replies to certain questions. As surveys were completed and submitted, each respondent's information was automatically entered into a secure and protected database, accessible only by the UIC NRTC project staff. The survey website and database were hosted with WebSurveyor Corporation, a private, for-profit research firm. All transmitted data were encoded using Secure Sockets Layer encryption. Neither Internet Protocol (IP) addresses linked to specific hardware used to complete the survey, nor any other identifying information about the respondents were collected. All research procedures were reviewed and approved by the University of Illinois at Chicago Institutional Review Board.

Inclusion and Exclusion Criteria

Individuals eligible to be included in the study were those who self-identified as having experienced mental health difficulties. The recruitment advertisement used for the study began as follows:

> "We are conducting a survey of people who have used mental health services or have experienced emotional or mental health problems. We would like to know how much control they have over their lives and important life decisions, such as where they live, what kind of work they do, and how they spend their money…" (Web Survey Advertisement).

Again, when they logged onto the survey website, read the informed consent material, and consented to participate in the study, respondents were instructed on the first page of the survey as follows:

> "[This] survey is about the experiences of adults (age 18 and older) who have used mental health services or have experienced emotional or mental health problems...By participating in this survey, you are helping to inform the mental health field about self-determination. Only adults who have used services or experienced mental health difficulties should complete this survey..." (Web Survey Instructions, p.1)

It was felt that these two ways of informing individuals about the study's intended target population would be adequate but perhaps not sufficient to ensure participation of only the intended respondents. Thus, near the end of the survey, participants were asked a number of questions about their psychiatric histories, mental health-related groups with which they identified, and their current relationships with service providers. These questions were examined to determine whether survey participants were indeed members of the target population of the research, and serve as the source of data analyzed in the present study.

Exclusion criteria included individuals who could not read English, those without access to the Internet, individuals who did not self-identify as mental health consumers, and minors (given human subjects requirements of parental consent, all information from individuals indicating that they were less than 18 years of age was excluded). The survey was posted for 9 months from July 2003 through April 2004.

Survey Instrument

The Web-based survey was programmed using a "dynamic" or interactive format (Tourangeau, 2004) and included automated skip patterns, immediate range and error checks, forced responses to all applicable items, and respondent-generated data submission. Some of the survey items were adapted from those used by the U.S. Bureau of the Census in its Technology Survey (Neuburger, 2001), as well as items from the Pew Internet and American Life Project survey protocols (Fallows, 2000). Other items were created by the UIC NRTC Web Survey Project Workgroup. The survey was comprised of three basic sections: 1) a section asking respondents about the degree of self-determination in their lives; 2) a section asking about their access, use, and barriers regarding information technology; and 3) questions about demographic characteristics and clinical history. A draft version of the survey was field-tested and revised according to psychometric results and field-test respondents' feedback. The present analysis used data from the survey's first and third sections.

Analysis

After inspection of frequency distributions and descriptive statistics, chi square and t-test analysis were used to explore demographic and clinical characteristics of those with different self-identifications. Following that, the mean self-determination scores of individuals with different self-identifications were examined and tested for differences.

Results

Survey Completion and Response Rates

The first research question was whether Web survey technology would reach individuals with psychiatric disabilities and how they would respond to attempts to recruit them into a survey on self-determination. Given the use of convenience sampling, it was impossible to determine the number of eligible individuals who were contacted during the recruitment phase of the study, but decided not to complete the survey, the typical definition of a refusal rate. However, WebSurveyor technology did enable us to determine the number of times the survey was "requested," that is, the number of times the survey was called up from the WebSurveyor server by a browser. Of the 1741 times the survey was requested, 1042 respondents completed the instrument and clicked on the "submit" button. This ratio suggests a response rate of 60%. However, it is possible that some respondents who did not submit the survey on the first try returned to request, complete, and submit it at a later date. Due to human subjects considerations, researchers did not capture the Internet Protocol (IP) address of respondents' computers, which would have enabled us to answer this and other questions about whether the survey was requested or submitted from the same computer on multiple occasions. However, the Web survey approach does appear to have been successful in recruiting a large number of research participants whose disabilities are both hidden and accorded a great amount of social stigma.

Because the survey was intended for respondents age 18 or older, which was also mentioned in the survey advertisement, a screening question early in the protocol itself asked whether they were under this age. Respondents answering in the affirmative were immediately directed to a "Thank you" page, which expressed the researchers' gratitude for their willingness to participate, but explained that they did not meet study eligibility criteria and ended the survey. However, in 11 instances, individuals' responses to this and a later follow-up question about age indicated that they were legal minors and their data was not included in the analysis, further reducing the study N from 1042 to 1031.

Respondents' Self-Identification

The next research question was how respondents identified themselves in relation to their mental health and emotional difficulties. First, they were asked whether they were a consumer, survivor, client or user of mental health services or a person with emotional difficulties, all of which are terms commonly used in the various mental health recovery communities. In what follows, these individuals are referred to as people with "mental health problems." The large majority, 95% (n=981), checked this item, indicating that they were currently experiencing such problems or had in the past. Next, respondents were asked whether they "currently" had a "mental health service provider," as a means of identifying all those who were receiving mental health services at time of survey completion. One again, a sizeable majority, 83% (n=853), indicated the presence of a service provider in their lives. Finally, an item asked respondents whether their "mental health problems" currently kept them "from participating fully in work, school, housework, or other activities." Those who reported functional limitations due to their mental health problems were considered to have a "psychiatric disability." A lower proportion, 65% (n=675) responded "yes" to this item than to the first two, which was expected given that not all individuals experience role impairment as a result of their mental health difficulties. Other individuals reported their mental health difficulties by checking one of four items asking about hospitalizations for psychiatric reasons, receiving a diagnosis of mental disorder, taking psychiatric medications, or having had mental health problems as children.

In addition to the foregoing, however, there were seven respondents who did not indicate membership in any of the four groups and did not check any of the four items described above. Thus, they did not identify as having current or past mental health problems, were not receiving mental health services, did not experience functional limitations, had never been given a diagnosis, had never been hospitalized, and had no childhood age of onset to report. Closer inspection of their responses to a checklist item asking about other types of mental health stakeholder roles revealed the following self-identifications: two said they were relatives of someone with mental illness; a third reported being a service provider, a fourth checked both family member of someone with mental illness and program director/manager/supervisor categories; a fifth checked both teacher and student; a sixth checked government official, program director, and service provider; and the seventh individual checked a number of categories (family member, program director, researcher, student, advocate, employer, and service provider). Because they did not meet study inclusion criteria, these seven cases were removed from the data, so that the final study N used in the remainder of the analysis was 1024.

Demographic Characteristics of the Respondents

The next research question was whether respondents' demographic features varied according to their self-identified mental health status. Table 1 presents the demographic characteristics of the 1024 remaining eligible respondents according to their membership in each of the three categories described above.

Compared to the first two categories, smaller proportions of those with psychiatric disability were married or cohabiting (34% vs. 37-38%). Similarly, lower proportions those with disability were working (43% vs. 50-51%). The same was true for working full-time, reported by lower proportions of those with disability (25%) than those receiving services or having problems (33-35%). Compared to the other two groups, those with psychiatric disability also had the highest proportion of co-occurring disabilities (40%) and annual incomes under $15,000 per year (38%). Finally, they were older on average (45 vs. 43 years of age).

However, the three groups were highly similar on other characteristics. Just over three-quarters of all three groups were women (76%), the majority were Caucasian (85-87%) and had high school degrees (98%), and over half were college graduates (58-61%). Around a third (35%) of all three groups resided in urban areas, two fifths (40-41%) in suburban, and a quarter (23-25%) in rural areas.

Table 1 also presents the results of chi-square and t-tests in which members and non-members of each of the three groups were compared. Those with mental health problems were more likely than those not in this group to be female, Caucasian, and to have incomes below $10,000 and $15,000 per year; they were also less likely to be male, Hispanic, African American, minority, married, employed full-time or working at all, and have annual income greater than $50,000. Those currently receiving services were more likely than those who were not to be female, less likely to be African American or minority, less likely to be male or be married, to work or work full-time, and to have high annual income. Finally, those with psychiatric disability were less likely to be married, have a college degree, work or work full-time, and have high annual income; those with psychiatric disability were also more likely to be low-income and were older on average. Overall, membership in these three groups indicated more social and economic vulnerability due to lower income, education, employment, and lack of a spouse or intimate partner. Moreover, those with functional limitations stemming from their mental health problems appeared to be the worst off in these life areas.

Table 1. Demographic Characteristics of Individuals with Different Mental Health Problem Identifications

	Person with Mental Health Problems (N=981)	Current Mental Health Service Recipient (N=853)	Person with Psychiatric Disability (N=675)	Total (N=1024)
	%	%	%	%
Gender				
Female	76*	76**	76	75
Male	24*	24**	24	25
Race/Ethnicity				
Caucasian (not Hispanic)	87**	86	85	86
African-American (not Hispanic)	2*	2*	3	2
Hispanic	3**	3	4	4
Minority	6**	6*	7	7
Married/Living as married	38**	37**	34***	39
Education				
High school graduate	98**	98	98	98
College graduate	61	61	58**	62
Current Work Status				
Employed full-time	35***	33***	25***	37
Employed at all	51***	50***	43***	53
Annual Household Income				
Less than $10,000	20*	20*	22***	19
Less than $15,000	32**	32**	38***	30
Greater than or equal to $50,000	25***	25*	21***	27
Geographic Area				
Urban	35	35	35	35
Suburban	42	42	40	42
Rural	24	23	25	23
Mean age in years	43	43	45***	43

* = $p<.05$, ** = $p<.01$, *** = $p<.001$ in chi-square and t-tests comparing members and non-members of each group

DIFFERENCES IN CLINICAL CHARACTERISTICS

Next, respondents' clinical characteristics were examined and tested to explore any differences. As shown in Table 2, the three groups were highly similar in their proportions ever hospitalized for mental health reasons, ever hospitalized for substance abuse, having a diagnosis, taking psychiatric medications, and average age at onset of mental health problems. The only difference between the three groups was a higher proportion of co-occurring “other” disability among the group with psychiatric disability, compared to the other two groups.

Table 2. Clinical Characteristics of Individuals with Different Mental Health Problem Identifications

	Person with Mental Health Problems (N=981) %	Current Mental Health Service Recipient (N=853) %	Person with Psychiatric Disability (N=675) %	Total (N=1024) %
Ever hospitalized for mental health reasons	73***	70***	73***	68
Ever hospitalized for substance use reasons	13*	13	14*	12
Ever diagnosed with mental disorder(s)	100***	95***	96***	94
Ever taken psychiatric medications	100***	97***	98***	94
Other disability currently limits life activities	32	32	40***	32
Mean age experienced first mental health difficulties	18***	19	18***	19

* = p<.05, ** = p<.01, *** = p<.001 in chi-square and t-tests comparing members and non-members of each group

Comparing members of each category with non-members, those with mental health problems were more likely than those without to have been hospitalized for mental health and substance abuse problems, to be diagnosed with a mental disorder, and to take psychiatric medications; they were also younger at the onset of psychiatric illness. Those currently receiving services were more likely than those not to have been hospitalized for mental health problems, to have been diagnosed, and to take psychiatric medications. Finally, those with disability were more likely to have been hospitalized for mental health or for substance abuse problems, to be diagnosed with a mental disorder, to have taken psychiatric medications, and to have a co-occurring disability; they were also younger at the time of their illness onset. Overall, membership in these three groups indicated more co-occurring problems (such as substance abuse and other disabilities), and more clinical involvement (younger age at problem onset and history of taking psychotropic medications). Clinically, those with disability due to their mental health problems appeared to be worse off in only one of these areas – the presence of a co-occurring disability.

DEGREE OF PERSONAL SELF-DETERMINATION

The final research question was whether respondents' self-assessed level of self-determination differed according to their membership in each of the three groups. As defined in the survey instructions, the concept of self-determination referred to the freedom to be in charge of one's own life including one's finances, place of residence, friends, and activities. It also meant having the resources to create a good life, make responsible decisions, and choose where and how one received services and support for mental health problems. After reading this definition, respondents were asked to rate their current level of self-determination as low through high using a scale from 0 to 10.

Table 3. Self-Determination Ratings of Individuals with Different Mental Health Problem Identifications (N=1024)

	Self-Determination Rating			
	With this Identification Mean (Median)	Without this Identification Mean (Median)	ANOVA F Test	Kruskal-Wallis H Test Chi-Square
Person with Mental Health Problems	6.7 (7.0)	7.1 (8.0)	3.54 ns	7.78 **
Current Mental Health Service Recipient	6.6 (7.0)	7.1 (8.0)	6.49 *	8.38 **
Person with Psychiatric Disability	6.0 (6.0)	8.0 (8.0)	193.68 ***	187.11 ***
Total	6.7 (7.0)			

ns = not significant, * = p<.05, ** = p<.01, *** = p<.001

Table 3 presents mean and median self-determination ratings for members versus non-members of each of the three groups. Compared to those without mental health problems, those with these problems had lower mean and median self-determination scores. However, the Kruskal-Wallace chi-square test revealed a significant difference in medians but the ANOVA F test did not reveal significant differences in the distributions of these ratings. Both the chi-square and ANOVA were significant for those currently receiving mental health services; here, those receiving services had significantly lower mean and median self-determination ratings than those not receiving services. Finally, those who reported functional impairment or disability related to their mental health problems had significantly lower mean as well as median self-determination ratings compared to those without disability. Thus, overall, membership in each of the three groups was associated with lower levels of self-assessed self-determination.

SUMMARY AND CONCLUSIONS

The results of this study revealed that Web survey technology was successful in reaching and recruiting a large number of individuals with mental health problems to participate in a research study of self-determination. However, several important challenges in using this survey methodology to study this group were also identified. First, even though the target population was clearly identified in both survey advertisements and in the introduction to the instrument itself, some individuals who completed the survey did not meet eligibility criteria and had to be excluded. Thus, it is critical in such surveys to include items that verify whether or not respondents have the appropriate characteristics and experiences to qualify them as members of the target population. Second, even among those who did meet inclusion criteria, there was a noteworthy degree of variability in self-identifications. Those with functional limitations, those receiving mental health services, and those with mental health problems were significantly different from their counterparts on demographic features, clinical characteristics, and level of self-determination. This highlights the diversity of this population and the related necessity of clarity on the researcher's part in defining and operationalizing the respondent pool.

Turning to the advantages and disadvantages of online recruitment and Web-based survey methodology in this study, several observations bear noting. First, this design yielded a very large sample of individuals from a specialized population that is highly stigmatized – people with significant mental health problems and impairments. Obtaining such a sample through traditional means would have been much more labor intensive and costly. Second, given the diverse self-identifications of this group, the interactive nature of the survey programming allowed administration of a protocol with complex skip patterns yet accompanied by very little respondent burden. For example, after reporting that they had a current service provider, service users were automatically directed to one set of questions about self-determination while nonusers were presented with another set. This and later skip patterns in the protocol would have been much more difficult for respondents to negotiate with a paper and pencil instrument.

On the other hand, there are concerns about the overrepresentation in this survey's respondent population of women, those with college educations, and Caucasians. While this was not surprising given that the last two characteristics mirror those of today's typical Internet user (Lenhart et al., 2003), it still calls for caution when interpreting the results. Still another concern was the fairly high level of self-determination reported by the study respondents in the face of a large volume of literature pointing to the low levels of self-determination among individuals with psychiatric disabilities. Perhaps self-determination is higher among Internet users, or among some sub-groups of individuals with severe mental illnesses. This possibility is supported by research suggesting that individuals who use the Internet are more likely than nonusers to feel that they have control over their lives (Lenhart et al., 2003). Unfortunately, our study design does not permit us to address these and other intriguing questions about respondent self-selection and resulting lack of sample representativeness. Thus, the tradeoffs found in prior Web-based survey studies conducted with a wide variety of populations were true of this one as well.

Overall, the results of this study suggest that self-determination among people with psychiatric disabilities is an important concept that can be fruitfully investigated using Web-based survey technology. However, caution must be applied by researchers using this approach given that respondents with different self-identifications have different background characteristics and clinical experiences and, most importantly, different levels of self-determination. Hopefully future research can build on study findings to explore correlates of both self-determination and self-identification among this group, enhancing the possibility for self-determination to become more fully realized. In this way, larger numbers of people with psychiatric disabilities can move toward the achievement of maximal independence and full participation in community life.

REFERENCES

Birnbaum, M.H. (2004). Human research and data collection via the Internet. *Annual Review of Psychology*, 55, 803-832.

Center for Mental Health Services. (1998, July). *Proceedings of the Midwestern United States Regional Consumer Meeting*. Kansas City Airport, Kansas City, Missouri.

Cook, J.A. and Jonikas, J.A. (2002). Self-Determination Among Mental Health Consumers/Survivors: Using Lessons from the Past to Guide the Future, *Journal of Disability Policy Studies*, 13(2), 87-95.

Cook, J.A., Hoffschmidt, S., Cohler, B.J., and Pickett, S. (1992). Predicting marital satisfaction among parents of offspring with severe mental illness living in the community. *American Journal of Orthopsychiatry*, 62, 552-563.

del Vecchio, P., Fricks, L., and Johnson, J.R. (2000). Issues of daily living for persons with mental illness. *Psychiatric Rehabilitation Skills*, 4(3), 410-423.

Epstein, J. and Klinkenberg, W.D. (2002). Collecting data via the Internet: The development and deployment of a Web-based survey. *Journal of Technology in Human Services*, 19(2/3), 33-47.

Fallows, D. (2000). *The Internet and daily life*. Washington, DC: The Pew Foundation.

Fawcett, J.F. and Buhle, E.J. (1995). Using the Internet for data collection. *Computers in Nursing*, 13, 273-279.

Gonzalez, J.E. (2002). Present day use of the Internet for survey-based research. *Journal of Technology in Human Services*, 19(2/3), 19-31.

Im, Eun-Ok and Chee, W. (2002). Issues in protection of human subjects in Internet research. *Nursing Research*, 51(4), 266-269.

Im, Eun-Ok and Chee, W. (2004). Issues in an Internet survey among midlife Asian women. *Health Care for Women International*, 25, 150-164.

Joinson, A. (1999). Social desirability, anonymity, and Internet-based questionnaires. *Behavior Research Methods, Instruments, and Computers*, 31(3), 433-438.

Kraut, R., Olson, J., Banaji, M., Bruckman, A. Cohen, J. and Couper, M. (2004). Psychological research online: Report of the Board of Scientific Affairs' Advisory Group on the Conduct of Research on the Internet. *American Psychologist*, 59(2), 105-117.

Lenhart, A., Horrigan, J., Rainie, L., Allen, K., Boyce, A., Madden, M. and O'Grady, E. (2003). *The ever-shifting Internet population: A new look at Internet access and the digital divide*. Washington, DC: The Pew Internet and American Life Project.

Murray, D.M. and Fisher, J.D. (2002). The Internet: A virtually untapped tool for research. *Journal of Technology in Human Services*, 29(2/3), 5-18.

Neuburger, E. (2001). *Home computers and Internet use in the United States: August 2000.* Washington, DC: U.S. Department of Commerce, Bureau of the Census.

Ranchhod, A. and Zhou, F. (2001). Comparing respondents of email and mail surveys: Understanding the implications of technology. *Marketing Intelligence and Planning*, 19(4), 254-262.

Rothman, J., Smith, W., Nakashima, J., Paterson, M.A., and Mustin, J. (1996). Client self-determination and professional intervention: Striking a balance. *Social Work*, 41(4), 396-405.

Rosenfield, S. (1991). Homelessness and rehospitalization: The importance of housing for the chronically mentally ill. *Journal of Community Psychology*, 19, 60-69.

Subramanian, A.K., McAfee, A.T. and Getzinger, J.P. (1997). Use of the World Wide Web for multisite data collection. *Academic Emergency Medicine*, 4, 811-817.

Tower, K.D. (1994). Consumer-centered social work practice: Restoring client self-determination. *Social Work*, 39(2), 191-196.

Tourangeau R. (2004). Survey research and societal change. *Annual Review of Psychology*, 55, 775-801.

United States Department of Education. (2000, May 18). Federal Register, Volume 65, No. 97.

Ware, N.C. and Goldfinger, S.M. (1997) Poverty and rehabilitation in severe psychiatric disorders. *Psychiatric Rehabilitation Journal*, 21(1): 3-9.

In: Towards Best Practices for Surveying People..., Volume 1 ISBN 1-60021-195-X
Editors: Thilo Kroll, David Keer et al., pp. 47-69

Chapter 4

USING AMERICAN SIGN LANGUAGE IN ASSESSING THE END-OF-LIFE-CARE EDUCATIONAL NEEDS OF DEAF PERSONS: LESSONS ON LANGUAGE, CULTURE, AND RESEARCH PRACTICES

Barbara Allen[1], Nancy Meyers, John Sullivan, and Melissa Sullivan
Carleton College Department of Political Science, Northfield, MN

ABSTRACT

This chapter reports on a community-based participatory research (CBPR) strategy for collecting health related data from a linguistic minority in the United States: self-identified members of the Deaf community. The meager literature available on deaf and hard of hearing persons' health and healthcare status suggests that these individuals rarely participate in government surveys of citizens' well-being. Culturally identified Deaf individuals, moreover, often view researchers from the "hearing world" with suspicion. Using CBPR and ASL-GLOSS (an American Sign Language—ASL—linguistics method), trained Deaf interviewers asked 130 Deaf senior citizens who depend on a signed language for communication questions about cultural practices and linguistic barriers to healthcare, focusing on end-of-life care information.[1] Interviews were videotaped and a centrally located monitor received direct feeds from five enclosed interview booths. A mirror placed behind the respondents enabled interviewer and respondent to be captured on the same videotape. The closed-ended questions of the half-hour interviews were coded on-site by the Deaf interviewers for statistical analysis. A team of Deaf interviewers reviewed the tapes to check the reliability of the initial coding and to assign categories and codes to open-ended questions. A focus group comprised of expert Deaf interviewers, community leaders, and hearing researchers reviewed and interpreted the findings. The survey instrument and method revealed important findings concerning deaf senior citizens' perceptions about their end-of-life care needs, enabling the development of appropriate educational materials and information dissemination

[1] Contact Information: Barbara Allen ballen@carleton.edu, Department of Political Science Carleton CollegeNorthfield, MN 55057 507-6464117

strategies. The research team concluded that the conceptual, sociocultural, and linguistic challenges of culturally identified deaf and hard of hearing persons can be addressed using CBPR strategies and ASL-GLOSS linguistic methods. These innovations in survey design and method can have a significant impact on collecting valid and reliable data from this underrepresented population.

INTRODUCTION: THE LESSONS INSPIRING COMMUNITY-BASED PARTICIPATORY RESEARCH

In 1999, eight Deaf and two hearing Minnesotans established the leadership team of *The End-of-Life Care Education Project of the Minnesota Deaf Community* (the Project).[2] The team's aims included training Deaf hospice volunteers and producing linguistic and culturally appropriate end-of-life care educational materials for Deaf people and their families. The tremendous response of health care professionals and Deaf families to the Project's activities underscored not only this population's need for access to information and services but also the educational needs of professionals charged with providing services for this community. Several experiences in hospice care settings revealed barriers to communication: Project-trained volunteers encountered Carl, whose brain injury made his signing legible to only those whose first language was American Sign Language (ASL); the volunteers also met Clara, a ninety-year-old woman who was the only Deaf resident at her care facility, cutting her off from all social intercourse. In Carl's case, communication barriers brought humiliation until Deaf volunteers explained to caregivers that his small gestures were in fact the ASL sign for "toilet" (Allen et al. 2002). In Clara's case, Deaf volunteers were able to show that Clara's lack of communication was not a manifestation of dementia, but an artifact of the linguistic isolation of a lucid elderly adult, with limited English literacy skills and a cultural reluctance to confide in a hearing person (a hospice chaplain).

Anecdotal reports suggested other significant obstacles to healthcare and information, including, for example, caregivers who relied on a Deaf patient's hearing family members for interpreting, not realizing that their patient might withhold important information about symptoms, rather than risk embarrassment (see also Committee on Disabilities of the Group for the Advancement of Psychiatry 1997) or find that a family member may be reluctant to pass on difficult news. Differences within the deaf population—age of on-set of deafness, residential school experience versus mainstreaming and a variety of communication preferences—further indicated the complexity of addressing the informational and care needs of the Deaf community. As Project team members considered the formal assessment of Deaf senior citizens' needs for health and end-of-life care information, it seemed clear that to generate reliable, valid, and useful knowledge, members of the community could benefit greatly by collaborating with and using the expertise of academics, in this case social scientists. Members of the Deaf community initiated the collaboration, making it all the more critical that Deaf people be involved in all aspects of the study—from constructing linguistically and culturally appropriate questions to interpreting results.

---

[2] We use the lowercase *deaf* when referring to the audiological condition of not hearing, and the uppercase *Deaf* when referring to a particular group of Deaf people residing in the United States and Canada who share a culture, use sign language as their primary means of communication among themselves, and hold a set of beliefs about themselves and their connection to the larger society (Padden and Humphreys 1988).

COMMUNITY-BASED PARTICIPATORY RESEARCH

Community-based participatory research (CBPR) begins by acknowledging the community as an aspect of collective and individual identity (Israel 2000; Israel, Parker, and Becker 1998). Indeed, in response to our question in Figure 1, our study found that a majority of Deaf seniors (65%) see themselves as "Deaf" first and as members of the United States polity second. Other principles of CBPR include: building on the organizational strengths, relationships, social structure and other resources of the community/culture; collaborating as partners in all phases of research (iterative processes of design, data collection and analysis); and creating opportunities for co-learning and empowerment in the interpretation and dissemination of results.

The next question is about how you identify yourself, or what you call yourself.

WHICH YOU WANT IDENTIFY YOURSELF? WHICH FIRST DEAF, SECOND AMERICAN.
FIRST AMERICAN, SECOND DEAF, WHICH?

	N	% Responding
1. Deaf American	80	65
2. American who is deaf	36	30
3. "R" sees no difference	6	5
Missing	3	
Total	125	100

Figure 1: Primary Identity

Community-based research (CBR) has revealed important cultural differences related to healthcare, a first step in increasing the relevance of research, identifying intervention strategies and adopting "best practices" within studied communities. By adding *participation* to the CBR philosophy, researchers in diverse communities have not only furthered these aims, but also enhanced trust and mutual respect among community members, researchers, and health professionals. CB*P*R has been shown to empower community members, enabling them to redirect their resources toward educational and action programs designed to promote well-being in their community. (CDC 1997; Hall 1992; Schulz, et al. 1998.).

In sum, CBPR partnerships join participants with diverse skills, knowledge, and expertise to address complex problems (Butterfoss, Goodman, and Wandersman 1987; Hall 1992; Himmelman 1992). Our experience suggests that CBPR played a vital role in collecting and interpreting data as well as in disseminating educational materials based on study findings. The sustained commitment of the researchers and Deaf community members in implementing "best practices" has produced subsidiary partnerships among Project team members, local institutions of higher education, Deaf (and hearing) hospice volunteers and practitioners, health care providers, and Deaf individuals and their families (see also Israel, Schurman, and Hugentobler 1992).

HEALTHCARE RESEARCH AND THE DEAF COMMUNITY

Nearly 23 million people (9.35% of the population) in the United States are categorized as having a hearing loss; approximately 4.8 million of these individuals cannot hear or understand speech (Adams, Hendershot and Marano 1999, Table 62, p. 93; Barnett 1999; Harmer 1999, Tamaskar et al. 2000). For those who are pre-lingually deaf and many others for whom deafness resulted from disease or injury at an early age, signed language is the primary mode of communication. Following Spanish, American Sign Language (ASL) is the second most commonly used minority (non-English) language in the United States (Barnett 1999); researchers estimate that at least two million Americans use ASL for everyday communication (Zieziula 1998). Although ASL represents the first language of a sizable number of Americans, there is no national database on deaf and hard of hearing (D/HOH) persons and little reliable data on the demographics, morbidity, or mortality of the deaf population or the ASL language group. For example, a recent examination of data sources of potential value for assessing the health and healthcare status of D/HOH on Medicare raised serious doubts about the reliability of the Medicare Current Beneficiary Survey (MCBS); 20% of people reporting a hearing loss in 1998 report normal hearing in 1999 and only 47% of people identified as deaf on the MCBS in 1998 also indicated that they remained deaf a year later (Delmarva Foundation and Gallaudet Research Institute 2002). The National Health Interview Survey (NHIS) records numbers of "hearing impaired" persons (Adams, Hendershot, and Marano 1999), but the survey does not distinguish the members of the distinct linguistic group—users of signed language—who are the focus of the present application.

The Deaf community is a unique languaculture (Agar 1994) whose members share a common language and history and participate in the formal societal structure of this distinct group (Becker 1980; Cohen 1995; Lane 1996; Lane 1993; Padden and Humphries 1988; Parasnis 1996; Sacks 1994). Research on this population's health and healthcare status remains extremely limited (Barnett 2002) and findings on medical care resource-use patterns are inconsistent (Delmarva Foundation and Gallaudet Research Institute 2002). Two results are remarkably uniform across all studies: 1) language differences raise a significant obstacle to the adequate care of Deaf individuals and 2) this population must be aggressively sought out and included in the national research agenda to improve the quality of healthcare for culturally diverse populations.

Differences in language and culture between the majority hearing population and Deaf people influence the healthcare provider-patient/client relationship (Barnett 2002b; Barnett 1999; Dipietro 1981; Ebert and Heckerling 1995; Harmer 1999; Lotke 1995; MacKinney et al. 1995; Shelp 1997; Solow 1981); may impede diagnostic and other aspects of healthcare provision for this linguistic minority (Harmer 2002; Iverson 2000; MacKinney et al. 1995; Steinberg, Sullivan, and Loew 1998; Zazove et al. 1993); and may significantly limit the Deaf individual's information on prevention and treatment of serious medical conditions (Baker-Duncan et al. 1997; Ebert and Heckerling 1995; Harmer 1999; Joseph 1995; Lass et al. 1978;

Tamaskar et al. 2000; Woodroffe et al. 1998; Zazove 1997; Zazove and Doukas 1994; Zazove et al. 1993). In the context of end-of-life care, language and cultural differences have an impact on the quality of end-of-life care and decision-making as well as bereavement counseling for dying persons who are Deaf, their family members, or Deaf persons who grieve the loss of family members, whether they are hearing or Deaf (Hines 2002; Zieziula 1998). The growing understanding of "health literacy"[3] also presents additional concerns for all cultural and linguistic minority populations—including members of the Deaf community. (Nielson-Bohlman, Panzer and Kindig 2004.) The combined forces of a vastly different language, the relative isolation of the community with undefined geographic boundaries, as well as cultural differences and limited health literacy present significant challenges in creating a data base of reliable, valid research. (Barnett 1999; Li et al. 2001).

Telephone surveys, while relatively inexpensive, under-represent this population (Barnett and Franks 1999) and, for reasons discussed at greater length below, self-administered (written) English questionnaires most likely will be unreliable. Yet the costs of interpreted interviews, translation and transcription to written English for the purpose of data analysis can be significant. Sampling also presents a research challenge, given the difficulties in identifying the portion of the population classified as D/HOH and the lack of registries for users of ASL, one indicator of affinity for the Deaf community. In many populations, the use of fortuitous samples (e.g. drawn from the membership of social organizations or responding to study advertisements) is generally acknowledged to introduce the potential for bias. Deaf clubs in towns and cities as well as national organizations draw from a highly networked population bound by residential school ties, highly subscribed local and national Deaf media, and annual national social and sports event gatherings (Becker 1980; Lane 1996; Lucas, Bayley, and Valli 2001; Padden and Humphries 1988; Parasnis 1996; Sacks 1994). Researcher biases—which can occur in instrument design, data collection and the interpretation of findings—may present an even more significant challenge than sampling bias for those who attempt to study this relatively closed community. A history of mistrust of hearing health professionals and academics compound the difficulties of research within this non-English language community (Barnett 2002b; Lane 1993; Li et al. 2001; Padden and Humphries 1988).

Beyond our experiences which led to the adoption of CBPR as a general research strategy, the reports of other researchers indicate three additional lessons for studies of Deaf individuals: 1) An interview protocol administered in person by a trained interviewer is preferable to a self-administered written survey or telephone interview; 2) Interviews should be conducted in the first language of the respondent (most often a signed language); 3) The benefits of fortuitous samples may mitigate the potential problems of bias. Further review of the literature on signed languages and Deaf culture suggests other factors affecting the researcher's ability to collect reliable data about Deaf people who use ASL as their primary mode of communication.

---

[3] According to the editors of *Health Literacy: A Prescription to End Confusion* the National Library of Medicine defines health literacy as: "the degree to which individuals have the capacity to obtain, process, and understand basic health information and services needed to make appropriate health decisions." See Nielsen-Bohlman, Panzer and Kindig 2004, 4.

SIGNED LANGUAGE AND DEAF CULTURE

In addition to the many anticipated challenges posed by language differences in cross-cultural studies, the linguistics of ASL raises several unique issues for researchers (Allen et al. 2002; Barnett 2002a; Barnett 2002b; Zazove 1997). ASL is a visual language whose signs are not adequately represented in written form (Baker-Shenk and Cokely 1991; Valli and Lucas 2002). The structure and grammatical characteristics of ASL are independent of English (Liddell 1980); *American* Sign Language designates the name of a language used by Deaf persons in North America, not (as is commonly believed) the signed equivalent of English. ASL provides no immediate or general access to the English language or any other spoken language.

The acquisition of English or another spoken language is extremely difficult for people who cannot hear (Hansen 2002). For most pre-lingually (and, depending on the individual's age of onset of hearing loss, many post-lingually) Deaf persons, English remains a second language (Caprici et al 2002; Liddell 1980; Lotke 1995; Moores 1997); average English reading levels for Deaf Americans have hovered around the fourth-grade equivalent for several decades (Holt, Traxler, and Allen 1997; Livingston 1997). As a result, the use of written English language questionnaires and other written modes of English-based communication between Deaf and hearing individuals are potentially unreliable. Questions phrased at the fourth-grade reading level may fail to reflect adequately the cognitive sophistication and depth of experience of Deaf respondents and question translation may be inconsistent across ASL interpreters. More significantly, important differences in the language, including the lack of homonyms, non-equivalence of metaphor, simile, and idiom, and the representation of some parts of speech (e.g. pronouns) by spatial references rather than signs, may give ambiguous meaning to *validated* English-language measures (Baker-Shenk and Cokely 1991). For example, anecdotal evidence reveals the depth of such problems in the contemporary example of the misinterpretation of the multiple meanings of the English term "positive," which leads Deaf individuals to understand their HIV+ status as a beneficent sign of health (See also Barnett 2002a).

Inconsistent interpretation of English constructs only increases the potential for data collected in English to be invalid or unreliable. Written questionnaires or ASL interpreted English-questionnaires that have been pre-tested on a Deaf sample may be adequate for the cost-effective measurement of some constructs (e.g. self-reported health habits such as smoking and alcohol use, number of visits to the doctor annually, and demographic data) (Lass et al. 1978; Tamaskar et al. 2000; Zazove et al. 1993), but a more complete picture of Deaf persons' experiences, beliefs, attitudes, and behaviors related to healthcare and end-of-life care may well necessitate multi-method approaches consisting of qualitative indicators and quantitative measures utilizing ASL (MacKinney et al. 1995; Witte and Kuzel 2000) and, for some constructs, Deaf interviewers and focus-group facilitators (Allen et al 2002).

The unique language, values and history of Deaf culture imply not only that construct validity, but also the accurate interpretation and acceptance of findings may depend on the continuing participation of members of the Deaf community in all research agendas. Unlike other minority languacultures, the Deaf community is often pathologically defined, an issue that continues to provoke distrust of medical professionals among individuals who define themselves as members of a distinct cultural minority (Lane 1993; Padden and Humphries

1988). In contrast to individuals who become deaf or hard-of-hearing later in life, many pre-lingual deaf individuals do not express their Deaf identity as a deficiency or the condition of deafness as a loss or lack. Rather, they present Deaf identity as one of the myriad distinct possibilities for the human being and, indeed, no data suggest that the lives of Deaf persons are less fulfilling than those of other (hearing) communities (Barnett 2002a; Barnett 2002b; Committee on Disabilities of the Group for the Advancement of Psychiatry 1997; Sacks 1994; Zazove 1997). Our study confirmed these findings and provided additional information about the residential school experience, socialization, and barriers that continue to impede access to adequate health information.

Most Deaf seniors in our sample created lifelong bonds with their residential school cohorts maintaining friendships that transcend geographic separation. In contrast, they shared a common language with neither their hearing parents nor, in most cases, their hearing siblings (Allen et al. 2002; Lane 1993; Padden and Humphries 1988). Ninety-five percent (a statistic that has remained remarkably consistent) of all deaf children are born to hearing parents showing similar results for our sample) many of whom do not learn ASL. Our sample population responded similarly (see Figure 2). For similar reasons, Deaf culture, thus, differs in how it is transferred among its members. Unlike other cultures, the language, norms and values of Deaf culture are transferred from peer to peer ("horizontally") instead of intergenerationally ("vertically") from parent to child (Barnett 2002a; Becker 1980; Committee on Disabilities of the Group for the Advancement of Psychiatry 1997; Parasnis 1996. Sacks 1994). Whether it is Deaf children with hearing parents or Deaf parents with hearing children, horizontal transference of culture presents significant issues for end-of-life caregivers and practitioners, including who is defined as "family."'

		N	% Responding
4. Attended Residential School	Yes	113	91.1
	No	11	8.9
TOTAL		124	100.0
5. Both parents hearing	Yes	117	94.4
	No	7	5.6
TOTAL		124	100.0

Figure 2: Residential School Attendance and Parents' Hearing Status

As Figure 2 shows, a significant portion of our sample population lived in residential schools, some up to 14 years. Most students returned home to their family of origin only at holidays severely limiting opportunities to participate in many family rites and rituals, including those related to death. Indeed, these respondents' views of "family" inclined to friends who shared the formative experience of Deaf residential school culture, rather than the biological tie generally understood by the majority culture as the basis of kinship (Allen et al. 2002; Becker 1980). The residential school experience influenced not only patterns of socialization, but also changed the individual's understanding and orientation to healthcare practices and information. Separation from the family of origin limited this population's access and understanding of such basic information as family medical history—indeed, anecdotal evidence indicates that in many cases, linguistic barriers prevented these Deaf seniors from knowing their own medical history (Allen et al. 2002; Barnett 1999; Clark 1995). As other studies have shown, children may not learn the causes of their illnesses when they do not share the language of their adult caregivers. Examination of residential health education curricula and preventive care instructions given by parents (or teachers) who do not use ASL also suggests that information may be limited to behavioral commands, without reference to the rationale for a given action (e.g. "brush your teeth," omitting the reason, "so you don't get cavities") (Clark 1995).

In addition to the language and cultural differences that distinguish this languagculture from other diverse populations is the lack of exposure to "incidental information"—news passively received by overhearing conversations, radio or television in the course of mundane activity. Lack of access to this kind of information, which plays a significant role in a person's ability to gather and analyze new concepts and ideas, generally is not accessible to Deaf persons, placing them at an even greater disadvantage when compared with their hearing counterparts. These factors—the lack of a common language and, in most cases, the cumulative experiences shared across generations with the family of origin as well as the inaccessibility of incidental information—have a profound affect on a Deaf persons' store of background knowledge. The existence of a sign for "background knowledge" illustrates the degree to which this reality is recognized within the broader Deaf community. The understanding of this concept (confirmed by the existence of a sign) stands in stark contrast to the lack of a sign for "hospice" or "advanced directive"—concepts not understood prior to the development of workshop materials and videotapes resulting from our research. The lack of background knowledge and access to information created a system of peer learning to fill information gaps, generating extensive networks that may amplify as well as correct misinformation (Becker 1980). Our findings suggested two related results: 1) gaps in background knowledge must be addressed before concepts relevant to end-of-life care can be made wholly intelligible and 2) the Deaf communication network is a highly evolved, sophisticated medium into which new information may be introduced (Allen et al. 2002).

Finally, the visual quality of ASL makes face-to-face communication essential, further encouraging the extensive relational networks at the core of the culture. Not only practical information, but also the literature and history of this culture are conveyed primarily in settings that allow for face-to-face interactions. Technological changes, including telecommunication devices (TTY/TTD) and e-mail, have enhanced rather than supplanted the cultural value of these networks. For all of these reasons, the norms of this "relational culture" must play an important role in the design of end-of-life care research. We believe that by addressing the unique characteristics of this population through a CBPR strategy, we have developed prototype research instruments that will allow other researchers to discover reliable and valid knowledge about the Deaf community in the healthcare setting.

Hearing individuals may not immediately grasp the profound difference between acquiring a spoken language by hearing the language and relying wholly on learning a language in its written form. ASL is acquired naturally; concrete experiences and abstract concepts are transmitted with the immediacy of a spoken language (Capirci et al. 2000; Lucas, Bayley, and Valli, 2001; and Washabaugh, Woodward, and DeSantis 1980). Nevertheless, the task of composing a grammatically correct English sentence without the benefit of modeling by hearing conventional usage requires additional skills that must be painstakingly acquired (Gallaudet Research Institute 1996; Gray 1956; Hansen 2002; and Holt, Traxler, and Allen 1997). Depending solely on English for communication with Deaf individuals invariably increases the probability of misunderstanding and stress.[4] Deaf elderly patients are not cognitively impaired, nor do they have limited life experience or suffer from an inability to communicate all the subtleties of emotion and ideas about their experience—in their own language. They will, however, like most of us, have difficulty communicating the full range of experiences very well in a second language. In that the Deaf individual may need to attain English proficiency to function in the hearing world, that hearing world has an ethical obligation to address barriers to communication in the healthcare setting.

ILLUSTRATIVE IMPLICATIONS FOR RESEARCH AND CARE

A brief summary of some of the key elements of the language will illustrate the depth of the issues Deaf people, researchers and healthcare professionals may encounter when communicating with one another. ASL, in summary, is a nonlinear language using space, facial expressions and hand and body movements, fully exploiting the capacities of vision, spatial relations, and visual-kinetic memory for storing and processing concurrent layers of information (Lane, Hoffmeister, and Bahn. 1996, 91). Facial expressions, "non-manuals," convey meaning. They include adverbs and information about sentence structure and organization. Linguists have identified over 250 grammatically governed facial expressions in ASL. Yet while these signifiers may be described, they involve subtle movements of face, tongue, eyes, eyebrows, lips, and mouth, and cannot be represented as written symbols.

ASL also displays grammatical elements such as the actors and objects of actions spatially. By pointing to a space(s) in front of the signer's body, the signer is able to use spatial arrangements to carry complex meanings that would require a lengthy text or explanation, if the same information were to be conveyed in a spoken or written language. The location of the sign relative to the body also carries information and can change the meaning of the sentence—including signs for "past," "present" and "future." An individual communicating her/his "pain" would perform that sign in the location where the pain occurs. Locating the sign by the temple for example, would indicate the individual has a headache.

Whether it is for purposes of conducting survey research or assessing pain, a very basic understanding of the linguistics of ASL can be instructive and increase one's appreciation for why some research with this population has produced unreliable data. A brief example illustrates the linguistic rule that signifies and distinguishes interrogative from declarative statements. "Yes/No" questions must be marked by raised eyebrows; "Wh-questions" (what, where, when, why and how) must be indicated with eyebrows down. To ask the question, "do you have any pain?" with eyebrows down is not only grammatically incorrect it may make some communication confusing. A recent study of the neurological controls of facial expressions of Deaf signers confirms two distinct functions of facial expressions—affective and linguistic. (Corina, Bellugi, Reilly, 1999.) Now consider the "Faces Pain Rating Scale," (Figure 3) a visual scale that often is used to help healthcare providers assess a patient's level

---

[3] The Project conducted three focus groups in which participants viewed three closed-caption videotapes about end-of-life care. Participants unanimously agreed that the English language usage was an obstacle to their learning about healthcare information.

and type of pain (Herr 2002; Herr 1998; Herr and Garland 2001; Herr, Mobily, Richardson, and Spratt 1997; and Wong and Baker 1988). The intent of the Faces Pain Rating is affective and in ASL has no linguistic association with pain (Herr 1998).[5] Rather, the linguistic function of the facials illustrated in Figure 3 are co-occurring facials used with the signs for happy, glad, surprise, depressed, sad, and cry (Costello 1994)[6].

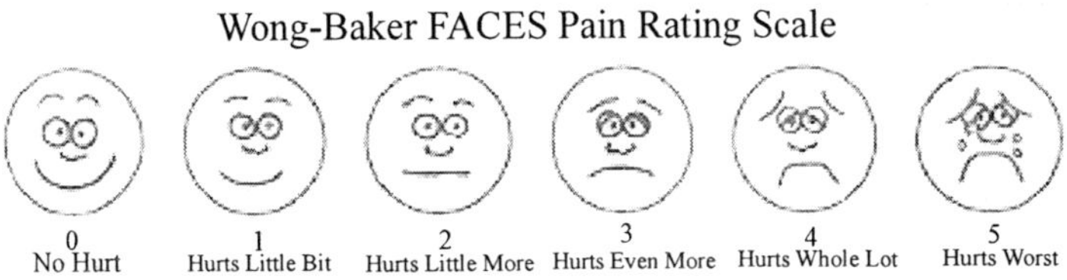

Figure 3

Numeric Pain Rating Scales (NRS), another popular pain assessment tool, rank orders pain numerically along a horizontal continuum that is typically graded as an interval measure ranging from zero to five, arrayed from left to right according to English language reading conventions. This spatial orientation has no meaning in ASL, where such ordering bears no connection to gradations of measurement, but often carries other meanings that convey depth and detail in the essentially non-linear narrative form of the language. We will address similar difficulties with Likert scales later in this chapter.

Mindful of the centrality of facials to ASL, we asked a few Deaf adults to tell us their opinion about probable results in using the Faces Pain Rating Scale (FPRS) with members of the ASL linguistic community. The results of this informal survey suggested that Deaf people, particularly individuals who are more vulnerable or with low reading literacy, might find the facials confusing. When symbolic faces are used in print to convey sentiments, they carry another set of meanings. Since humor, and teasing cannot be communicated and understood by voice, Deaf people often use words [(smile) or (haha)] parenthetically in the body of their TTY or e-mail messages and have adopted a series of keystroke conventions to convey specific affects. In fact, in one edition of a widely circulated national Deaf newspaper, *Silent News,* the entire back page was devoted to the keystrokes used to make a variety of "smiley faces." This range of "faces" seems to have found a place within the culture unrelated to any associations with the somatic conditions of pain.

Difficulties in communication pose similar difficulties in collecting data and disseminating information within the Deaf community. Our goal of obtaining a representative national sample required that the vast majority of the Deaf seniors be able to comprehend and answer our questions accurately. The only way to achieve this goals was to administer surveys

---

[5] Comparisons of various scales including the faces pain scale (FPS) (horizontal) numeric rating scale (NRS) given below, vertical visual analog scale (VAS), verbal numeric scale (VNS) and verbal descriptor scale (VDS) show that the age does not significantly effect the use of the FPS. Higher levels of pain were reported using the VNS and the VDS discriminated best between increasing intensities of pain. The VAS was subject to higher failure rate, as was the NRS when administered repeatedly in short periods of time.

[6] These scales are among the pain assessment tools made available to palliative care providers on many websites, including *Partners Against Pain* as cited, http://www.partnersagainstpain.com, accessed 5/10/02 and the American Medical Directors Association, http://www.amda.com/clinical/chronicpain/pain-face.html, accessed 5/15/02. Although neither organization recommends the use of this scale in groups other than those intended by Wong and Baker (1988), it has increasingly been accepted for use with adults under palliative care.

in ASL—*in their own language*—thereby allowing our Deaf respondents to communicate the subtleties of emotion and ideas about their experience. Beyond the question of language proficiency lie other issues, including cultural differences, which language holds in the deep recesses of interpretation and meaning.

Social scientists find that respondents often try to accommodate the researcher, giving what the respondent perceives as the popular, appropriate, or desired answer to a question. In cross-cultural research this particular bias is increased, especially if respondents are of a minority culture or language group—or simply perceive themselves to differ from the enculturated assumptions displayed by the researcher, research instrument, or research methodology. In cross-cultural research it is always preferable to use the native language of the respondents, if one hopes to gather accurate information about respondents' preferences, attitudes, and behaviors. We maintain that continuing to approach users of sign language with written English surveys will continue to produce results that contain significant inaccuracies.

Community-Based Participatory Research within the Deaf Community

In addition to technical and ethical concerns about language and facility with English, we were also aware of cultural differences that influence our findings as well as the care and education of the Deaf elderly. Language and culture are necessarily connected, as anthropologists have shown (Agar 1994, 60). The "Deaf experience" of our sample population was profoundly influenced by the residential school experience and subsequent outcomes that is central to aspects of Deaf culture.

One such outcome of the residential school was noted in anthropologist Gaylene Becker's 1976 pioneering study of Deaf seniors. Becker found that her respondents developed a peer learning process as "a formalized mechanism for coping with the information vacuum" (Becker 1980, 66-67). Peer learning is unlikely to address the individual's lack of family medical history, however, and it may not be a reliable source of public information, including news about health issues. As Becker also notes, information reliability is desirable, but difficult to maintain. As she explains, when stories are incomplete, people speculate; in any community, when the data do not add up, people bring as much coherence to the matter as they can, but rumor and misinterpretation often abound. On-going access to information is crucial to correcting misperceptions and, more importantly, preventing the amplification of errors in peer learning networks. Such earlier research findings played an important role in our efforts to assess the needs of the Deaf elderly for end-of-life care information.

To summarize this overview of research as it relates to our study, we conclude that self-administered English language questionnaires will be less effective in collecting reliable data than interviews conducted by Deaf interviewers in ASL. Furthermore, available research suggests that translations of English language questionnaires by non-native ASL users are likely to be ineffective in capturing the subtleties of cultural differences between members of the Deaf community and hearing ASL interpreters. Finally, existing research on suggests that members of the Deaf community must be an integral part of all phases of research if we hope to collect and interpret data reliably.

Many researchers do not fully understand or accept the points we have made about the inappropriateness of using English questionnaires with Deaf populations. At one presentation of our study to palliative care providers, a physician in the audience suggested that he could use a written English questionnaire and get the same results we did only far more efficiently. A second suggestion was to administer a written English questionnaire with an interpreter present to interpret anything the respondents indicated was not clearly understood. Unfortunately, research on ASL and the Deaf community suggests that this second approach tends to compromise the reliability of the interviewing process, because each question and concept needs to be signed in the same way for all respondents—a requirement unlikely to be met, as we learned in our experience with the Deaf community. Moreover, cross-cultural research also confirms the limitations of linguistic translations that fail to mediate the cultural divide that accompanies the differences in the languages of researcher and respondent. Hence, we developed a strict protocol of translation, from English to ASL, and ultimately, to ASL-GLOSS, described later.

THE STUDY

Overview

On September 12–14, 2001, 130 Deaf senior citizens attending the Deaf Seniors of America (DSA) conference participated in 30-minute interviews about their experiences and issues related to end-of-life care. The probability sample was drawn from the DSA list of 1000 registered conference participants. Invitations that included a form for scheduling an interview during the conference were mailed to the participants. Potential participants were contacted by fax, TTY, or email (according to their preference) to remind them of their appointments. These invitations, which were added to the general DSA conference mailing, confused some conference attendees, generating multiple contacts with the randomly selected group and their peers. News of the study spread quickly throughout the national networks of the Deaf community and we soon had a significant number of "volunteers" who contacted us, hoping to be interviewed. Subsequent volunteer recruitment proved vital to the project when the events of 11 September made it impossible for about half of the probability sample to attend the conference. Individuals participating in the interviews represented 33 states and all regions of the United States. Initial statistical analysis of the data show no significant differences related to our study's objectives between the probability sample and the volunteers. Key demographic information was collected from a self-administered English language questionnaire prior to the interviews. Answers to these questions were validated throughout the depth-interviews conducted in ASL by the fourteen Deaf interviewers, who we had recruited and trained in two, three-hour sessions where they learned research protocol and interviewing techniques. In addition to the majority of respondents who used ASL as their primary means of communication (97 respondents, 80 percent of the sample) about a fifth of the randomly selected respondents indicated their preference to have the study administered another signed language when they returned their study registration cards. The final respondent pool included twenty-eight individuals who requested that their interview be administered in Conceptually Accurate Signed English (CASE), the Rochester method (emphasizing finger spelling), or the Oral method, which incorporates speech and speech reading (Solow 1981). Members of the interview team accommodated these requests as well as the needs of one deaf/blind individual who had been randomly selected for the sample.

Interviews ranged from 30-40 minutes and covered nine topics: (see Figure 4.) 1) English reading and media use; 2) information dissemination; 3) obstacles to receiving information; 4) experiences with healthcare, especially communicating with a doctor; 5) end-of-life care and hospice; 6) decision making; 7) death and Deaf culture; 8) the Deaf community and 9) Deaf self-identification. Interviewers coded responses to closed-ended questions during the interviews. The one hundred twenty-eight interviews were recorded digitally and on VHS (two respondents declined to be videotaped) in five enclosed interview areas set up in a meeting room at the conference hotel.

Categories of Questions	
1.	Reading
2.	Where people get information
3.	Obstacles in getting information
4.	Communication with doctors
5.	End-of-life care and hospice understanding
6.	Decision making
7.	Death and Deaf culture
8.	Aspects of Deaf community
9.	Self-identification

Figure 4

A video monitor, placed in the center of the room received direct feeds from each of the cameras that recorded activity in the interview booths. This technology allowed us to switch among booths to monitor interviews and identify and address problems. A long mirror placed next to the respondent allowed the camera to capture both the interviewer signing questions and the respondent signing an answer (Figure 5). This set-up enabled us to capture questions and answers as a check on consistency, interviewers' use of discretionary probing questions, and problems or concerns with question wording in order to confirm interviewer reliability. Interviewers also coded responses to the questions during the interviews providing data for preliminary analysis. A complete review of the data required a detailed content analysis of the videotaped interviews, based on content categories generated in focus group discussions held with members of the Deaf community who are uniquely qualified to interpret the respondents' narrative explanation of their answers to our questionnaire.

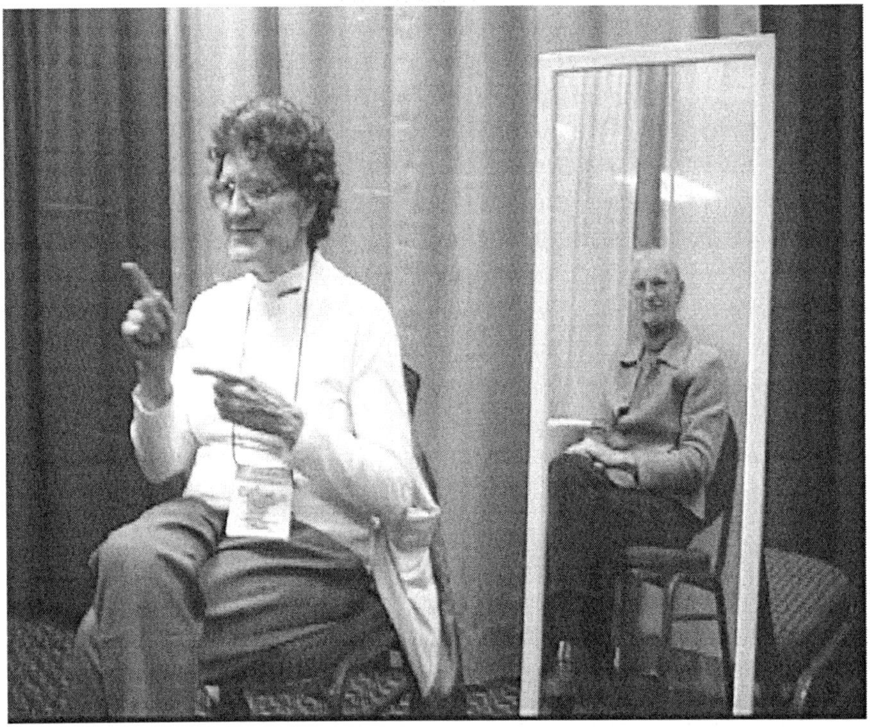

Figure 5.

USING CBPR TO DEVELOP THE QUESTIONNAIRE

From their experience with patients like Carl and Clara, mentioned earlier, The Minnesota Deaf End-of-Life Care Project team learned that they needed more information about the population they serve: How could the Deaf elderly best gain access to end-of-life care educational materials? What did the Deaf elderly know about this topic? What did they believe they needed to know? The Project team engaged two hearing social scientists to discuss the principles of CBPR and collaborate with members of the Deaf community to design a questionnaire and undertake the study.

Using standard survey research techniques, the principal investigators designed an English language interview schedule using validated measures of constructs when such questions were available. Leaders in the Deaf community (selected because of their years of experience in the Deaf community, participation in Deaf organizations, or their occupational expertise) discussed and revised the interview schedule in individual consultations and focus group settings. These sessions helped identify oppressive or intimidating questions, confusing question wording, and questions that reflected "English" cultural assumptions that were inappropriate to the Deaf cultural experience.

Some changes were surprising; for example, standard media use items failed to give reliable responses, and even the apparently straightforward question: *How much do you understand when you read the newspaper?* overestimated reading comprehension. One of our Deaf consultants explained that we must first ask which sections of the newspaper the respondent had read (headlines, sports, news stories, etc.), otherwise we might measure only that the respondent understood some proportion of the comics or the headlines. After more than a dozen iterations of critique and revision two pre-lingually Deaf University professors were trained in interviewing techniques and the survey tool was pre-tested on a small sample of Deaf seniors.

Following further revision of the instrument, one of the interviewers was selected to sign the questions and create a practice videotape. At this stage of the instrument design phase, the researchers became aware of the wide latitude interviewers might have in interpreting, translating, and signing the English questions. Concerns with interviewer reliability (signing the questions consistently) were first addressed by use of the model videotape. A lead Deaf interviewer met with the other thirteen interviewers to describe how to use the model tape as a guide in preparing for administering the interview schedule. The interviewers included linguists, teachers of ASL at the elementary, secondary and post-secondary level, Deaf ministers, and other professionals for whom ASL was their native language.

During the interviewer training sessions, these individuals also functioned as a focus group to determine question wording after the research team explained the intent and objective of each question. In these discussions it became clear that the linguistics of ASL would have a tremendous impact on all levels of our research. Even with agreement on question wording, disagreements about the specific signs that best represented the intended meaning of the question and the inflection to be used in distinguishing the intervals enumerated on the Likert scales remained. Scientifically reliable responses required the interviewers to reproduce the scalar intervals consistently; the content validity of the intervals, thus depended entirely on the consistent presentation of the non-manual adverbial markers of ASL. Despite initial skepticism about the reliability of these "facials," the investigators observed and accepted that their place in the linguistic structure of the language are no different than English grammar rules that govern the use of adverbs and adjectives. Decisions about the use of particular signs were made by the now-expert interviewers through consensus (a cultural preference for decision-making). Nevertheless, the significant differences between spoken and written languages and a visual, manual, and spatial language raised doubts about the effectiveness of the training video in ensuring the survey's reliability.

GLOSSING: THE KEY TO SUCCESSFUL INTERVIEWS

Although we believed we had faithfully recorded in English the back-translation of our experts' final decisions in ASL, in truth, we had failed. The interviewers worried that the translations represented on the training video were open to alternative interpretations and, indeed, they generally failed to render the English into a consistent set of signs. Our next step, also unsuccessful, was to engage the assistance of a bi-lingual (but culturally Deaf) senior citizen to write simple English sentences in ASL word order omitting the parts of speech that do not exist in ASL. Although we were moving in the right direction, our interviewer team found our representation of the ultimately unintelligible, if perhaps amusing. Our interviewer focus groups reminded us that there is no written form of ASL, suggesting that we use ASL-GLOSS to represent ASL equivalents of English. The representation of English in GLOSS required advanced linguistics skills available to only a few of our Deaf consultants or interviewers. ASL was not recognized as a legitimate language until the late 1960's, making it unlikely that many deaf people would have learned such a skill or, in many cases, even the rudiments of ASL grammar and syntax. One of our younger, more recently educated interviewers had the GLOSS skills we needed. Ultimately, GLOSS, the unique ASL linguistic method for translating and transcribing the cognitive equivalent of an English word or phrase, allowed for the reconstruction of the interview schedule in a uniquely "Deaf" final form.[7]

GLOSS is defined as English word or words used to represent a particular ASL sign in its most common meaning. GLOSS is not a written form of ASL, rather it represents common English equivalents of ASL signifiers (Valli and Lucas 2002). Although post-secondary schools, (e.g. Gallaudet University) teach this linguistic method and GLOSS has recently been introduced in primary grades as an aid to English language writing instruction (Mozzer-Mather 1990), "translating" from English to GLOSS is an advanced skill. Deaf interviewers with advanced degrees in ASL and linguistics understood the role that GLOSS could play in addressing the challenges that the investigators faced. Though most Deaf people do not have the linguistic skills to change English to GLOSS they had no difficulty reading GLOSS and signing it as written. GLOSS, in its complete form, represents all aspects of ASL (facial expressions, indexing or referring to a person or object spatially and body or role shifting.) Different use of any of these ASL grammatical markers can completely change the meaning and intent of a sentence. A signer, using the exact signs for TODAY RAIN, PICNIC CANCEL can change the meaning of this sentence by adding the co-occurring facial, "eyebrows up." With no facial, the sentence reads, "It's raining today, and the picnic is cancelled." With eyebrows up, the meaning changes to "If it is raining today, the picnic is cancelled." (Corina, Bellugi, Reilly 1999.) The Deaf interviewers however, felt that because of their intense participation in interpreting the meaning and intent of the questions, reading GLOSSED sentences written in BOLD uppercase English would be sufficient—it was not necessary to grammatically diagram co-occurring facial expression and manual signs. The GLOSS method proved to be the methodological discovery—a breakthrough resulting from the collaborative research approach—that addressed the threats to the study's reliability and validity by ensuring that the questions would be asked consistently in every interview.

THE ADAPTATION OF LIKERT SCALES

Likert scales are traditionally used to assess degrees of agreement or importance, as in "Do you strongly agree, agree, disagree, or disagree strongly with this [given] statement." As we observed in our discussion of pain analogue instruments, scalar representations ranging from left to right may not work effectively with ASL users, who more typically arrange degrees of measurement vertically and, in general, convey myriad meanings through a complex array of spatial orderings. Following the advice of a Deaf psychologist with whom we consulted, we changed the traditional horizontal scale to a vertical scale to accommodate ASL spatial reference points and non-linear attribute of ASL. Simply put, our consultant said, "everyone knows 'up' and everyone knows 'down.'" ASL also has its own numbering system. This does not mean that English numbers are not understood, it does, however, require that

[7] GLOSS represents the common English equivalent of an ASL signifier, or sign. For example, in the English question, "Should ASL interpreters be available for on-call emergency use?" the concept "on-call" was rendered in GLOSS as GO-GO-GO, meaning essentially, always ready to go or continually ready.

potentially serious ill Deaf patients "translate" a scale with numerals 1–5 below a line and facials above a line into a meaningful way to communicate their level of pain.

We encountered other problems in the conceptual response set for Likert scales, including the function of negation in ASL, especially the prohibited use of double negatives. Much like the English use of a rhetorical question—"You wouldn't want some ice cream, would you?"—as an affirmation, narrative conventions in ASL include the rhetorical use of negation to signal a speaker's desire for confirmation or agreement: an insidious source of bias to the unwary researcher. In ASL, double negation results in a nonsensical loop of "cancelled" meanings, compounding the problem of interpretation. For our research, ASL convention required us to recast scale categories so that, for example, "Not very important" became *IMPORTANT LITTLE* and "Somewhat important" became *SO-SO*. After reading the ASL question, the interviewer prompted respondents using 8 ½" x 11" cards showing numbered scalar categories, a device suggested by one of the interviewers that greatly facilitated the speed and ease of interviewing. The scalar categories appeared in GLOSS on one side of the card and English on the other side, giving the interviewer flexibility in accommodating literacy skills of Deaf interviewees.

Questionnaire Layout

Our 22 page survey went through fourteen complete revisions, including revisions to the layout that improved the visual accessibility of the instrument. Interviewers had 30 minutes in which to ask 64 questions and code responses. To facilitate the administration of the questionnaire by people who rely solely on visual cues, we formatted the entire survey in two columns and color-coded sections (See Figure 6). The topics of each section (which appeared earlier in Figure 2) were represented in green. The English version of the question (black) was followed by the GLOSSED version in bold uppercase. Short instructions to guide the interviewers were in red, while the scalar representations appearing in the second column were in blue. The Likert scales appeared in written English followed by a GLOSSED version of the scale. Ultimately, every aspect of the survey instrument was designed to accommodate the demands of a visual, manual language. From the color coding and page layout, to adaptations of the Likert scales and the use of ASL-GLOSS, our questionnaire reflected the collaboration of hearing researchers and members of this distinct linguistic minority. The interviewer focus groups and instrument pretests confirmed the importance of the visually oriented, color-coded layout of the questionnaire presented in English and ASL GLOSS. As noted in the Overview, recording the responses of Deaf seniors also reflected our method for accommodating the requirements of a visual language.

TOPIC # 3 – QUESTIONS ABOUT OBSTACLES IN GETTING INFORMATION I will ask you questions about obstacles/frustrations in getting health information.	
⇒ Deaf people have different preferences for communication. What is your preference? **12. DEAF PEOPLE HAVE PREFERENCE COMMUNICATION, DIFFERENT, DIFFERENT, DIFFERENT. YOUR PREFERENCE, WHAT?** (sign list in right column ⇒)	**ASL** **Signed English** **Lip reading** **Fingerspelling** **Other**
⇒ How important is it for you to get **health information** in the way you prefer? 12. YOU PICK ________**(repeat response above)** NOW YOU-TELL-TO-ME UNDERSTAND HEALTH INFORMATION, HOW IMPORTANT USE? HOW IMPORTANT? (sign list in right column ⇒)	1. Very important 2. Important 3. Somewhat important 4. Not very important 5. Not at all important **1. VERY IMPORTANT** **2. IMPORTANT** **3. IMPORTANT SO-SO** **4. IMPORTANT LITTLE** **5. NOT IMPORTANT**

Figure 6

CONCLUSION

This chapter highlights a cross-cultural research strategy for research in the Deaf community, suggesting how full participation of Deaf citizens as experts in their culture enable a research process designed to overcome cultural barriers to research, and potentially health knowledge. Using CPBR, we were able to engage the Deaf community's expertise to design a questionnaire and interview format that has allowed us to collect reliable valid information about Deaf seniors' end-of-life care knowledge, attitudes, preferences, desires, and experiences. Our study confirms that language and cultural differences matter, whether researchers are gathering data or care providers are disseminating healthcare information. Ninety-two percent of our respondents told us that they learn best when information is presented in a visual format and that complex information is most easily understood in a signed language; about ninety-four percent indicated that it was important that they receive health-related information in their preferred language. Deaf individuals who cannot access general information in their language cannot fully participate in meaningful conversations in the public arena of policy making, or, indeed, in many healthcare settings. Lack of access to health-related information raises important ethical and practical issues for healthcare and healthcare research.

The foundation of community-based participatory research assumes the full and active participation of citizens as experts in the research process. Our experience with CBPR confirms that the participation of members of the Deaf community enabled us to identify ethical dilemmas posed by linguistic and cultural differences as well as the impact the lack of background knowledge has on an individual's health literacy. The ethical issues implied by our results continue to emerge as we work with members of the Deaf community in focus groups designed to help us interpret our data. Thus far, it seems clear that visual media, ASL is the best way to convey healthcare information to the Deaf community.

Furthermore, our research experience suggests that Deaf people must be a part of the team charged with designing and presenting such instructional media. In this case, doing *with* rather than doing *for* a community is much more than a slogan. Collaboration may be the only approach that can bring members of the Deaf community the information they need to make informed, thoughtful decisions about their care; collaboration in developing intervention activities and strategies for practitioners who provide services for this unique languaculture may, likewise, be imperative.

REFERENCES

Adams, P.F., G.E. Hendershot, and M.A. Marano. 1999. Current Estimates from the National Health Interview Survey 1996. *National Center for Health Statistics*. Vital Health Stat 10 (200). Hyattsville (MD): U.S. Department of Health and Human Services Publication No (PHS) 99, 1528.

Agar, M. 1994. Understanding the Culture of Conversation. New York: William Morrow.

Allen, B., N. Meyers, J.L. Sullivan, and M. Sullivan. 2002. "Sign Language and End-of-Life Care: Research in the Deaf Community." Healthcare Ethics Committee Forum: *An Interprofessional Journal on HealthCare Institutions' Ethical and Legal Issues* 14 (3):197–208.

Baker-Duncan, N., J. Dancer, B. Gentry, P. Highly, and B. Gibson. 1997. "Deaf Adolescents' Knowledge of AIDS." *American Annals of the Deaf* 142 (5): 368–72.

Baker-Shenk, C. and D. Cokely. 1991. American Sign Language: *A Teacher's Resource Text on Grammar and Culture*. Washington: Gallaudet University Press.

Barnett, S. 2002a. "Cross-cultural Communication with Patients Who Use American Sign Language." *Family Medicine* 34 (5): 376–82.

Barnett, S. 2002b. "Communication with Deaf and Hard-of-Hearing People: A Guide for Medical Education." *Academic Medicine* 77 (7): 694–700.

Barnett, S. 1999. "Clinical and Cultural Issues in Caring for Deaf People." *Family Medicine* 31 (1):17–22.

Barnett, S. and P. Franks. 1999. "Telephone Ownership and Deaf People: Implications for Telephone Surveys." *American Journal of Public Health* 89 (11): 1754–756.

Becker, G. 1980. *Growing Old in Silence*. Berkeley: University of California Press.

Breivik, E., A. Gudmundur, and E. Skovlund. 2000. "A Comparison of Pain Rating Scales by Sampling From Clinical Trial Data." *The Clinical Journal of Pain* 16: 22–28.

Butterfoss, F.D., R.M. Goodman, and A. Wandersman. 1993. "Community Coalitions for Prevention and Health Promotion." *Health Education Research* 8: 315–30.

Capirci, O et al. 2002. "Gesture and the Nature of Language in Infancy: The Role of Gesture as a Transitional Device En Route to Two-Word Speech." *In The Study of Signed Languages*, eds. D.F. Armstrong, M.A. Karchmer, and J.V. Van Cleve. Washington, DC: *Gallaudet University Press*, 213–46.

Center for Disease Control and Prevention (CDC) and Agency for Toxic Substances and Disease Registry. 1997. Principles of Community Engagement. Atlanta: *CDC Public Health Practice Program*.

Clark, J.K. 1995. "Health Education Curricula in Residential Schools for the Deaf." *American Annals of the Deaf* 140 (5): 410–14.

Cohen, L.H. 1995. Train Go Sorry: Inside a Deaf World. New York: Vintage.

Committee on Disabilities of the Group for the Advancement of Psychiatry. 1997. "Issues to Consider in Deaf and Hard-of-Hearing Patients." *American Family Physician* 56 (8): 2057–2064.

Corina, David P., Bellugi, Ursula, Reilly, Judy. 1999. "Neuropsychological Studies of Linguistic and Affective Facial Expression in Deaf Signers." Language and Speech 42 (2-3): 307–31.

Costello, E. ed. 1994. American Sign Language Dictionary. New York: Random House.

Delmarva Foundation for Medical Care, Inc. and Gallaudet Research Institute. 2002. Identification of Performance Standards for the Deaf and Hard of Hearing: Report on the Analysis of Data Sources for Assessing the Health Status of Deaf and Hard of Hearing People. Washington: *Gallaudet University Press*.

DiPietro, L.J., C.H. Knight and J.S. Sams. 1981. "Health Care Delivery for Deaf Patients: the Provider's Role," *American Annals of the Deaf.* 126(2):106–112.

Ebert, D.A., and P.S. Heckerling. 1995. "Communication with Deaf Patients: Knowledge, Beliefs, and Practices of Physicians." *Journal of the American Medical Association* 273 (3): 227-29.

Gallaudet Research Institute. 1996. Stanford Achievement Test, 9th Edition, Form S, Norms Booklet for Deaf and Hard-of-Hearing Students. Washington, DC: Gallaudet University.

Gray, W.S. 1956. *The Teaching of Reading and Writing: An International Survey*. Chicago: Scott Foresman and Co.

Hall, B. L. 1992. "From Margins to Center? The development and purpose of Participatory Research" *American Sociologist* 23: 15–28.

Hansen, B. 2002. "Bilingualism and the Impact of Sign Language Research on Deaf Education." In The Study of Signed Languages, eds. D.F. Armstrong, M.A. Karchmer, and J.V. Van Cleve. Washington, DC: *Gallaudet University Press*, 172–89.

Harmer, L.M. 1999. "Health Care Delivery and Deaf People: Practice, Problems, and Recommendations for Change." *Journal of Deaf Studies and Deaf Education* 4 (2): 73–110.

Herr, K. 1998. "Evaluation of the Faces Pain Scale for Use with the Elderly," *The Clinical Journal of Pain* 14: 29–38.

Herr, K. and L. Garland. 2001. "Assessment and Measurement of Pain in Older Adults." *Clinics in Geriatric Medicine* 17 (3): 457–78.

Herr, K. as reported at http://www.nursing.uiowa.edu/research/news/elderpain, accessed 5/10/02.

Herr, K. P. Mobily, G. Richardson, and K. Spratt. 1997. "Pain Intensity Assessment: Use of Experimental Pain to Compare Psychometric Properties and Usability of Selected Scales in Adults and Older Populations." *Presented at Annual Conference of the Pain Society*, New Orleans.

Himmelman, A.T. 1992. Communities Working Collaboratively for a Change. Minneapolis: Humphrey Institute of Public Affairs, University of Minnesota.

Hines, S.K. 2002. "The Unique Bereavement Counseling Needs of the Deaf and Hard of Hearing." *The Thanatology Newsletter* 8 (1): 6–9.

Holt, J.A., C.B. Traxler, and T.E. Allen. 1997. Interpreting the Scores: A User's Guide to the 9th Edition Stanford Achievement Test for Educators of Deaf and Hard-of-Hearing Students. *Gallaudet Research Institute Technical Report* 97-1. Washington, DC: Gallaudet University.

Israel, B.A. 2000. "Community-Based Participatory Research: Principles, Rationale and Policy Recommendations." Address, National Institute of Environmental Health Services, Division of Extramural Research and Training Meeting on Successful Models of Community-Based Participatory Research, Washington, DC.

Israel, B.A., E.A.Parker and A.B. Becker. 1998. "Review of community-based research: Assessing partnership approaches to improve public health." *Annual Review of Public Health* 19: 173–202.

Israel, B.A., S.J. Schurman and M.K. Hugentobler. 1992. "*Conducting Action Research:* Relationships between Organization Members and Researchers." *Journal of Applied Behavioral Science* 28: 74–101.

Iverson, L. 2000. "Long-Term Care for Deaf Elders: Exploring Residential Options." *Geriatric Care Management Journal* 10 (4): 7–16.

Joseph, J.M. 1995. "Sexual Knowledge, Behavior, and Sources of Information Among Deaf and Hard or Hearing College Students." *American Annals of the Deaf* 140 (4): 338–44.

Lane, H., R. Hoffmeister, and B. Bahn. 1996. *A Journey into the Deaf-World.* San Diego, CA; 1996.

Lane, H. 1993. The Mask of Benevolence: Disabling the Deaf Community. New York: Vintage.

Lass, L.G., R.R. Franklin, W.E. Bertrand, and J. Baker. 1978. "Health Knowledge, Attitudes, and Practices of the Deaf Population in Greater New Orleans—A Pilot Study." *American Annals of the Deaf* 123 (5): 960–967.

Li, R.M., P. McCardle, R.L. Clark, K. Kinsella, and D. Berch. 2001. Diverse Voices—The Inclusion of Language-Minority Populations in National Studies: *Challenges and Opportunities*. Bethesda: National Institute on Aging.

Liddell, S.K. 1980. *American Sign Language Syntax.* The Hague, Netherlands: Mouton Press.

Liddell, S.K. 2002. "Modality Effects and Conflicting Agendas." *In The Study of Signed Languages*, eds. D.F. Armstrong, M.A. Karchmer, and J.V. Van Cleve. Washington, DC: Gallaudet University Press, 53–81.

Livingston, S. 1997. Rethinking the Education of Deaf Students. Portsmouth (NH): *Elsevier*.

Lotke, M. 1995. "She Won't Look at Me." *Annals of Internal Medicine* 123 (1): 54–57.

Lucas, C., R. Bayley, and C. Valli. 2001. *Sociolinguistic Variation in ASL. Vol. 7 of Sociolinguistics in Deaf Communities*. Washington, DC: Gallaudet University Press.

MacKinney, T.G., D. Walters, G.L. Bird, and A.B. Nattinger. 1995. "Improvements in Preventive Care and Communicatin for Deaf Patients: Results of a Novel Primary Health Care Program." *Journal of General Internal Medicine* 10 (3): 133–37.

Moores, D.F. 1997. "Psycholinguistics and Deafness." *American Annals of the Deaf* 142 (3): 80–88.

Mozzer-Mather, S. 1990. "A Strategy to Improve Deaf Students' Writing Through the Use of Glosses of Signed Narratives." *Gallaudet Research* Institute working paper 90–94. Washington: Gallaudet University Press.

Nielsen-Bohlman, L., A.M. Danzer and D.A. Kindig, eds. 2004. Health Literacy: *A Prescription to End Confusion*. Washington, D.C.: National Academies Preess.

Padden, C. and T. Humphries. 1988. *Deaf in America, Voice from a Culture.* Cambridge, MA: Harvard University Press.

Parasnis, Ila. ed. 1996. *Cultural and Language Diversity and the Deaf Experience.* New York: Cambridge University Press.

Sacks, O. 1994. Seeing Voices: A Journey Into the World of the Deaf. New York: Harper Collins.

Schulz, A.J., B.A. Israel, S.M. Selig, I.S. Bayer, and C.B. Griffin. 1998. "Development and Implimentation of Principles for Community-Based Research in Public Health." *In Research Strategies for Community Practice.* ed. R.H. Macnair. New York: Haworth Press. 83-110.

Shelp, S.G. 1997. "Your Patient is deaf, Now what?" *Registered Nurse.* 60(2):33–37.

Solow, S.N. 1981. Sign Language Interpreting: *A Basic Resource Book.* Silver Springs: National Association of the Deaf.

Steinberg, A.G., V.J. Sullivan, and R.C. Loew. 1998. "Cultural and Linguistic Barriers to Mental Health Service Access: The Deaf Consumer's Perspective." *American Journal of Psychiatry* 155 (7): 982–84.

Tamaskar, P., T. Malia, C. Stern, D. Gorenflo, H. Meador, and P. Zazove. 2000. "Preventive Attitudes and Beliefs of Deaf and Hard-of-Hearing Individuals." *Archives of Family Medicine* 9 (6): 518–25.

Valli, C., and C. Lucas. 2002. *Linguistics of American Sign Language.* 3rd ed. Washington: Gallaudet University Press.

Washabaugh, W., J.C. Woodward, and S. DeSantis. 1980. *Providence Island Sign: A context-dependent language.* Washington, DC: Gallaudet University Press.

Witte, T.N. and A.J. Kuzel. 2000. "Elderly Deaf Patients' Health Care Experiences." *Journal of the American Board of Family* Practice 13 (1): 17–22.

Wong, D.L. and C.M. Baker. 1988. "Pain in Children: A Comparison of Assessment Scales," *Pediatric Nursing* 14 (1): 9-17.

Woodroffe, T., D.W. Gorenflow, H.E. Mador, and P. Zazove. 1998. "Knowledge and Attitudes about AIDS among Deaf and Hard of Hearing Persons." *AIDS CARE* 10 (3): 377–86.

Zazove, P. 1997. "Understanding Deaf and Hard of Hearing Patients." *American Family Physician* 56 (8): 1953–954.

Zazove, P. and D.J. Doukas. 1994. "The Silent Health Care Crisis: Ethical Reflections of Health Care for Deaf and Hard-of-Hearing Persons" *Family Medicine* 26 (6): 387–90.

Zazove, P., L. C. Niemann, D.W. Gorenflo, C. Carmack, D. Mehr, J.C. Coyne, and T. Antonucci. 1993. "The Health Status and Health Care Utilization of Deaf and Hard-of-Hearing Persons." *Archives of Family Medicine* 2 (4): 745–52.

Zieziula F. 1998. "The World of the Deaf Community." In *Living with Grief*, eds. K. Doka and J. Davidson. Levitown, PA: Bruner/Mazel Publishers, 181–98.

In: Towards Best Practices for Surveying People..., Volume 1 ISBN 1-60021-195-X
Editors: Thilo Kroll, David Keer et al., pp. 71-87

Chapter 5

CONSUMER-DRIVEN AND CONDUCTED SURVEY RESEARCH IN ACTION

Jonathan Delman
Consumer Quality Initiatives, Inc.

ABSTRACT

A core flaw of mental health systems in the United Sates is the lack of consumer direction in research and intervention design. When mental health consumers play a significant role in research and evaluation activities, they are in a position to provide early consideration of the relevance of the research topic and advise on how findings can best be applied in their communities.

Consumer Quality Initiatives, Inc. (CQI) has offered a direct response to this problem. CQI is a mental health consumer-directed and staffed quality improvement and research organization based in Massachusetts. CQI's mission is to give consumers a greater voice and an integral role in evaluating their treatment and to initiate changes based on data collected. CQI's overall approach is based on the principles of Community-based Participatory Action Research ("CPAR").

CQI conducts much of its work through in person interviews and focus groups, then writing in depth data driven reports. The "personal" approach, as opposed to telephone interviews and written questionnaires, is critical because many mental health consumers distrust "the system," and they are less likely to open up to staff or student interviewers. Because of their personal experience with mental illnesses, CQI interviewers are able to build a rapport with respondents that help them speak honestly and openly about their treatment experiences.

People with disabilities are often seen as only the objects of survey research. Consumer Quality Initiatives, Inc. (CQI) is a consumer run research and evaluation organization that has attempted to turn this paradigm on its head. Below is a self-reported case study of CQI's methodology.

Statement of the Problem

The recent President's New Freedom Commission report (Achieving the Promise: Transforming Mental Health Care in America) is one highly critical of the nation's mental health system (Dept. of Health and Human Services, 2003). Among other critiques, the report concluded that the mental health service system has not been responsive to the needs of consumers and families, and that the findings of rigorous research have not been effectively translated into practice (DHHS, 2003, pp 67) (Institute of Medicine, 2001). Thus, a significant recommendation of the President's report is to involve consumers and families in the planning and evaluation of services, with a specific reference to consumer lead research and evaluation (DHHS, 2003, pp 37).

A core flaw of our mental health system is the lack of consumer direction in research and intervention design. When mental health consumers play a significant role in research and evaluation activities, they are in a position to provide early consideration of the relevance of the research topic and advise on how findings can best be applied in their communities. Consumers are in fact capable of taking a lead role in survey research, but only if they are provided with the resources to support training and infrastructure.

In particular, mental health consumer survey methodologies have not been effective in producing high quality data due to poor sample representations and lack of respondent openness. The consumer run personal interviewing apparatus, with its familiarity with the "community," is the critical component to developing a consumer driven system where relevant research is effectively translated into practice.

Historical Perspective

Historically, public mental health policy makers, system administrators, and program evaluators have not directly involved people with mental illness in systems planning and quality improvement efforts (DHHS, 2003, pp 27). In fact, it's likely that most of policy and research leaders did not see any value of including consumers in the developing research and evaluation projects, and thus never even considered it.

The report of the President's Commission notes that people with mental illness often experience stigmatizing attitudes from others. It may be that some systems planners and researchers have held discriminatory judgments/stereotypes that attach to people diagnosed with a mental illness. That is, people with this label are generalized to be cognitively challenged, lacking in judgment, unreliable, unpredictable, or any combination of the above (United States Public Health Service Office of the Surgeon General, 1999). However, studies now demonstrate that recovery is possible people with mental illness and that many with mental illness are contributing value to our society, for example taking on the roles of wage earners and parents (Harding, Brooks, et al, 1987a). In fact, there is a developing literature on the experience and expertise that people with mental illness bring to the table (Deegan,1993). Thus, a reliance by policy makers and researchers on stereotypes has reduced the value overall of their research and the policies developed.

The lack of participation of people with serious mental illness in policy-making is also related to their high rate of poverty, and frequent reliance on public assistance, including

Social Security and Medicaid (United States Public Health Service Office of the Surgeon General, 1999). Consumers are often unemployed and there is no mental health "consumer union," ie, something that binds them beyond their disability. Consumers thus lack the power of a purchasing unit, which ultimately provides a position at the policy table. That is, they do not have the purchasing power that comes with being and actual "consumer."

Thus, there has been no natural incentive for providers and brokers of these services, such as government and managed care companies, to market to or to partner with this disenfranchised group. Consumers of publicly funded services are provided with little, if any, information about their service options, and they do not receive training that would even allow them to use such information effectively. In effect, key decision makers have not seen the inherent market value of consumer direction.

Fortunately, attitudes and philosophies have begun to change, and it is now not uncommon for people who work in the mental health field to talk about recovery for people with mental illness (Harding, Brooks, et al, 1987a). There are several reasons for this, only a few of which I will mention. First, starting in 1970's, consumers began to organize on both a national and statewide level. Second, the federal government began to fund consumer organizing activities, and encourage such efforts on a local level.

In addition, the literature now favors a robust mental health consumer voice in the planning and evaluation of mental health services. Chaney has defined that voice as "meaningful participation in the design, delivery, and monitoring of health care" (Chaney, 2002). One important purpose here is to hold managed behavioral health organizations "accountable for the reasonableness of their practices" (Sabin, O'Brien and Daniels 2001). As stated in a recent working paper, consumer involvement needs to go beyond satisfaction measures to formally involve consumers in system design, implementation, and monitoring. To be meaningful, the participation has to be sustained over time and focused on crucial elements of the program. Consumers will only participate if they feel their voice has an impact. (Forquer and Sabin 2002).

During the 1990's, some consumer groups advocated local governments to help them determine the avenues by which consumers could use data to affect practice and policy. For example, in 1990, the city of Philadelphia provided funding for the establishment of the Consumer Satisfaction Team (CST) model. With this model, an independent organization run and staffed by family members and consumers, who interview service recipients about their services in a fairly informal way (Smith, 2000). Reports on providers are written by the organization and then shared with high level decision makers. Several cities and states followed suit, as Massachusetts did in 1999.

And in 2003, Recommendation 2.2 of the President's report stated clearly that the system must "Involve Consumers and Families in Planning, Evaluation, and Services":

> In the past decade, mental health consumers have become involved in planning and evaluating the quality of mental health care and in conducting sophisticated research to affect system reform. Consumers have created and operated satisfaction assessment teams, used concept-mapping technologies, and carried out research on self-help, recovery, and empowerment.

Local, State, and Federal authorities must encourage consumers and families to participate in planning and evaluating treatment and support services. The direct participation of consumers and families in developing a range of community-based, recovery-oriented treatment and support services is a priority.

The Massachusetts Experience- Precursor to CQI

The groundwork for a consumer satisfaction team approach in Massachusetts had long been laid by the consumer movement and its dedicated leaders. As part of this movement, a state-wide consumer-lead advocacy group called M-POWER opened its doors in 1987.

M-POWER, which stands for Massachusetts People/Patients Organized for Wellness, Empowerment and Rights, became concerned in the early 1990s when the state established a managed care behavioral health carve-out to manage the delivery of acute care services to people with serious mental illness, but did not involve consumers in any serious way in its development. With its attempts to get a seat at the table stymied, in 1997, M-POWER lead a protest march to the office of the Commissioner of MassHealth, which lead to regular meetings with key state officials.

In 1998, the mental health Medicaid carve out, MBHP[1], agreed to a performance incentive with the state Medicaid office by which it would contract with a consumer-run group that would interview clients about the quality of their programs, analyze the data, and write reports. In January 1999, MBHP contracted with M-POWER, which formed the Massachusetts Consumer Satisfaction Team Initiative (MCST) to carry out the contract terms. On April 28, 2000, this group established a separate corporate identity called Consumer Quality Initiatives, Inc., or CQI.

As a project of M-POWER, the work initially involved developing our own survey instruments, which would allow us to pinpoint areas of strength and weakness on the part of providers, with the hope of affecting systematic change, rather than simply placing blame. Some providers volunteered to participate, which allowed us to demonstrate our competence and value. Other providers then opened their doors, and those who did not were eventually required to do so by MBHP. Eventually, we received funding from the state Department of Mental Health (DMH) as well.

Consumer Quality Initiatives, Inc.

Objective

Consumer Quality Initiatives, Inc. (CQI) is a mental health consumer-directed and staffed quality improvement and research organization based in Massachusetts. CQI's mission is to give consumers a greater voice and an integral role in evaluating their treatment and to initiate changes based on data collected. A primary activity of CQI is to collect information by interviewing consumers and family members via a structured or semi-structured surveys and writing in depth data driven reports. The goal is to improve service quality and to transform a flawed system to one that is recovery oriented and consumer driven.

[1] Massachusetts Behavioral Health Partnership, a subsidiary of ValueOptions

Staffing

CQI is unique in that it is a research and evaluation organization that is run by community members, in this case people with mental illness.

CQI is consumer operated organization. According to its bylaws, at least 51% of CQI's board of directors must be, and are, mental health consumers. CQI's founding (and current) executive director is a mental health consumer, and its staff is made up of both consumers and family members. As such, all board members and staff have had some direct experience with the mental health system, and recognize that CQI exists to affect policy and practice, not simply to write reports for publication.

CQI has five full-time staff: executive director, director of operations, research coordinator, western Massachusetts coordinator, and research associate. CQI also hires a several part-time staff, some of whom have a particular expertise, such as our accountant and a data base expert. Others are hired on a more irregular basis, usually to conduct interviews, with CQI having about 5-7 active people to cover the Commonwealth (all full-time staff interview as well). Part-time work is advantageous for many who continue to receive benefits, such as Social Security disability, that have limitations on how many hours the recipient can work.

Funding

A majority of CQI's revenues are derived from two ongoing contractual arrangements. One agreement is with the Massachusetts Department of Mental Health (DMH), and a larger one is with the state Medicaid behavioral health managed care company, the Massachusetts Behavioral Health Partnership (MBHP). Most of the work here is quality improvement related, though needs assessments are conducted.

About one-third of CQI's revenues are derived from subcontracts they develop with universities and medical centers to lead qualitative evaluations of large mixed method research projects. These arrangements are often written into grants, and sometimes CQI is brought in after a grant is obtained.

A small amount of CQI's revenues are derived directly from private grants, and CQI has demonstrated success in grant activities. Yet, CQI has not been able to obtain grants in a manner earlier hoped.

A small amount of CQI's revenues are based on contracts with individual provider agencies to conduct quality improvement surveying. CQI also works with consumer organizations to train consumers about quality management. CQI also engages in general consulting on consumer measures and surveying, its clients including the federal Center for Mental Health Services and the Veterans Administration.

Business Model: An Independent 501(C) (3) Survey Research Organization

CQI's existence as an independent 501(c) (3) organization is critical to its success. CQI's mission is different from other consumer run organizations in that it does not provide services, advocate for individuals or organize consumers. Thus, CQI's being a project another organization would dilute its mission and challenge its objectivity.

In fact, many providers and other groups have valued our independence from state government and managed care companies. By not being part of government or a managed care company, we are not seen as being co opted for other purposes. Also, program clients in particular are more likely to open up to an independent group than to program staff.

The effective implementation of personal interview research on a large scale requires the focus of a single organization. The best research interviewers, consumer or not, use their skills on a regular basis, and confer with fellow interviewers to perfect their technique. CQI conducts a rigorous day and a half training for all new interviewers, and more experienced staff work with them in vivo until their skills are well developed. In addition, CQI provides strong quality controls through regular supervision, and review of interviewer notes or taped transcriptions. Review of an orally transcribed interview is a powerful method for providing interviewers with critical feedback, which can be ongoing as needed.

In addition, the practice of arranging and conducting personal interviews is an expertise that needs to be homed. CQI is in a position of quickly sizing up a situation and deciding how best to recruit respondents; what incentives, if any, to offer; and what information to give to and get from providers and authorities to help them recruit. Also important is an excellent knowledge of privacy, confidentiality, and legal protections --such as Internal Review Boards (IRBs) and HIPPA-- so that barriers to success are quickly removed.

Having collected data on different aspects of the Massachusetts mental health system during the last six years, CQI is able to make both geographic and temporal comparisons, and know the system well. Not only is CQI able to make quality improvement recommendations, but large-scale systemic recommendations (Delman, 2004).

Analytical Framework: Community-Based Participatory Action Research

CQI's approach is based on the principles of Community-based Participatory Action Research ("CPAR"), which is defined as a:

> collaborative process that equitably involves all partners in the research process and recognizes the unique strengths that each brings. CPAR begins with a research topic of importance to the community with the aim of combining knowledge and action for social change to improve community health and eliminate health disparities. (Minkler, Blackwell, Thompson and Tamir, 2003).

CPAR recognizes the community to be a unit of identity, and that a sense of community is cultivated by identification and emotional connection with other members (Israel, Schultz,

Parker, Becker, Allen and Guzman, 2003). A key characteristic of CPAR is the commitment to focus on and augment existing strengths and assets in a community.

A key feature of CPAR is that "the community" drives the research agenda (Israel et al, 2003). The involvement of the community in all phases of the research is necessary to ensure that professionals do not misconstrue or render meaningless information collected due to their lack "lived experience" or because they are not a member of that socio-cultural group. (AHRQ, 2004, Danley and Ellison, 1997). The participatory process thus assumes the legitimacy of consumer expertise produced outside of the scientific community, and looks to build on that expertise. (Gaventa,1993).

Community-based research methodologies equitably involve all stakeholders in the research process and recognize the unique strengths that each brings. Essential to community-based research is the active re-allotment of power between all involved members and constituents in the research process (Strand, Marullo, Cutforth, Stoeker, Donohue, 2003a). CPAR emphasizes reciprocal transfer of knowledge, skills and capacity throughout the process, imparting community members with tangible and practical benefits as a result of their engagement and participation (Springett, 2003). Thus, CPAR strengthens co-learning and capacity building among all partners.

In essence, the purpose of community-based research is not simply to develop knowledge within a discipline, but to create knowledge that "contributes to making a concrete and constructive difference in the world" (Sclove,1997, p. 542). This approach promotes innovation and improves quality:

> By being involved, participants can see the value of the information they are collecting. Involvement also ensures that the indicators are meaningful to all concerned. . . . However, the benefits of such an approach go beyond ownership and clarity. Involving a range of people in each stage often generates innovative ways of measuring process, impact, and outcomes. (Minkler and Wallerstein, 2003).

Involvement of community members establishes the critical link between research and action or practice because community members buy in to a process that involves them from the beginning and they are in a better position to apply findings to actual practice and disseminate those findings (Israel et al, 2003). CPAR is more easily translated into practice since community-defined research is relevant to the local conditions, with consumers taking an equal role (Israel et al, 2003). Consumers not only buy in to it, but can explain it to their peers.

CPAR aims for long-term and sustainable outcomes (Israel et al, 2003). CPAR disseminates findings and knowledge gained to all partners and involves all partners in this process (Israel et al, 2003). CPAR aims to achieve this with a heightened sensitivity toward presenting the information gained in language that is understandable and respectful to all partners involved. CPAR is dedicated to engaging in projects that can be sustained over time from one funding source to the next, as well as heartily acting in a way that translates findings to improved outcomes.

Despite skepticism from more traditional or conventional scientific communities, community-based participatory research has the necessary rigor and is valid and reliable (AHRQ, 2004, Simpson and House, 2002). A review of the research on the quality of community-based participatory action research reveals the high quality of these studies in the rigor of the design, increased participation rates, increased external validity, reduced attrition rates, and increased individual and community capacity (AHRQ, 2004).

The CPAR philosophy is critical for mental health transformation, where even the best research findings usually are not to be translated into routine practice for 15-20 years, especially with regard to "minority communities and other disadvantaged populations" (AHRQ, 2004, Institute of Medicine, 2001). A major reason for this disparity is that the community is not engaged in applying these efforts. The community has much expertise in understanding these issues, but little access to research design and implementation, let alone researchers who develop projects based on the expressed concerns of community stakeholders.

METHODOLOGY

CQI's methodology consists of a series of processes that are supported by a necessary infrastructure. The set of processes are at a minimum to: 1) develop or adapt surveys based on consumer expressed preferences, 2) conduct personal interviews or focus groups with clients/consumers, 3) analyze data and write reports with recommendations, 4) present reports to relevant stakeholders, and 5) develop action plan(s). Since the goal is to maximize the consumer voice in survey research, CQI's methodology requires that it lead and participate in every step of the research process. CQI's general mode is thus to lead a survey research project and act collaboratively with other research partners, or to not participate at all.

CQI's approach to survey research is considered more radical than other forms of CPAR since CQI is an organization of mental health consumers with strong ties to the grassroots, participates in survey research decision making, and aims for systems to make structural change, not just individual program change (Stoecker, 2003, Wallerstein and Duran, 2003).

INFRASTRUCTURE

The infrastructure for such a methodology requires that the processes be carried out by an organization that is not only consumer run (see above), but also has "full service" capacity, ie: to initiate and complete survey research projects. (CQI's full-service methodology contrasts with a partial service approach, by which an organization may work for a larger institution only to conduct interviews or only to advise on data interpretation.) This "full service" approach allows CQI, as the consumer run organization, to ensure that the consumer voice is represented throughout the research process, and not "watered down" at any one point. Lack of consumer direction at either the development of the research questions and measures, data collection, data analysis, or report dissemination will significantly diminish the value of that research to the community (Springett, 2003).

Another reason for the full service approach is to avoid tokenism, and further contributions to stereotypes held by academia and policy makers about consumer run organizations. Many funders are now looking at research applications that involve consumers with great favor. CQI has been approached on several occasions by academia to take on the role of hiring interviewers for a large research project. When so approached, CQI's response has been that its purpose is actually to influence the research process, so that it will not be "interviewers for hire."

In one case, an academic researcher, as part of grant application, wanted CQI staff to be interviewers for that institution, which would have provided the interviewer training, not CQI. CQI's response was that their expertise is to train interviewers and otherwise take leadership in a survey project. The researcher made clear that it was unwilling to give up control of any aspect of the research process, even interviewer training, to CQI, ie the community. CQI thus declined to participate and was not included in the grant application. In another case, however, the academic researcher who initially wanted to minimize CQI's involvement in the research process, decided to include CQI in a more significant way in the grant application, though this took much negotiation.

In addition, CQI could not build the necessary capacity to carry out its work on a statewide basis by taking on bit parts of other research projects. The costs of CPAR, and personal interviews in particular, are significant but not fully appreciated by funders and academia. Thus, the full service approach allows CQI to build capacity, to support operational costs (staffing being very significant as noted below) and the costs of CPAR development. CQI's adherence to CPAR principles requires that it develop research proposals and grant applications that reflect the expressed needs of consumers, not simply what a few people think is a good idea.

The sophisticated nature of personal interview survey research requires that CQI staff, made up of consumers and family members, be experienced in a variety of research areas (ie, consumer researchers and evaluators). Thus, three of the five main staff have advanced degrees, two in applied research. Over time, staff have developed a significant expertise in survey design, coordinating interviews, conducting personal interviews, and qualitative review. Where CQI staff does not have expertise, board members, friends, or consultants have been helpful. CQI's excellent track record as evaluators has brought us loyal clients and excellent feedback on the readability, comprehensiveness, and utility of the reports.

PROCESSES

Survey Development

CQI has developed a survey development approach that reflects the preferences of consumers and is respectful of the views of other stakeholders. This approach consists of the following: 1) a literature review, 2) establishment of a multi-stakeholder survey development work group which meets on semi-regular basis, 3) consumer focus groups, 4) drafting of survey, 5) cognitive lab interviews, 6) piloting of instrument, and 7) review with workgroup for instrument finalization.

This stage also provides CQI with the opportunity to develop a survey protocol. Considerations here include outreach to people eligible for interviews, role of incentives, location of interviews, and need for IRB approval.

Personal Interviews

The key to CQI's survey process is that personal interviews are used to collect data, and the interviewers are people in recovery from mental illness or family members.

Mental health consumer survey methodologies, which often rely on mail and telephone techniques, have not been effective in producing the high quality data due to poor sample representations and a lack of respondent openness (Holbrook, Green and and Krosnick, 2003). People with mental illness are oftentimes a "vulnerable segment of the population," and thus less likely to have phones or even get mail, particularly homeless people. And when responding by phone, this group tends to be less than candid in their responses, having a tendency to satisfice (Holbrook, 2003).

[D]ata obtained from telephone interviews appear to be more distorted by satisficing and a desire to appear socially desirable than are data obtained from face-to-face interviewing, and respondents interviewed by telephone are more suspicious and less motivated to optimize (ie., less cooperative and less interested in the survey (Holbrook et al, pp ,2003).

Also, respondents who have learned to distrust the system are less likely to open up to staff or student interviewers, as compared to consumers interviewers (Simpson and House, 2002). Because of their personal experience with mental illnesses, CQI interviewers are able to build a rapport with respondents that help them speak honestly and openly about their treatment experiences. This is part of the hard-earned expertise that consumers gain through as having been or being service recipient (Deegan,1993).

Mental health systems and programs have usually dictated to consumers how things will be run, with limited opportunity for input. As a result, most mental health consumers are not in the habit of thinking critically about the quality of their care. Program clients have sometimes been given written questionnaires to fill out, but many have not filled them out due to a lack of understanding of how they would be used, a lack of trust, and reading comprehension problems. And since the parameters of the questionnaires have been defined by non-consumers, consumers are not necessary given the opportunity to respond to questions that most matter to them. Interviews also help breach any reading comprehension gaps.

CQI interviews are conducted in private, and information that would identify the person interviewed is not shared with anyone[2]. Respondent then have an unusual opportunity to open up, and they are often stunned to the point that they are not ready to answer open-ended questions with much detail. However, CQI's interviewers are there to prompt them in a way to think thoughtfully and critically about the quality of their care. Thus, if asked how a program is helping them, respondents may shrug their shoulders or just say something like "groups." The interviewer's job is to sit with them for a moment, give them further time to think, and if they don't get an explanation, to ask why they say "groups."

Project Development

Critical aspects of a project's development are driven by the purpose of the survey research project. These aspects are described directly below, and examples of these processes are described in the Results section.

---

[2] Unless legally mandated.

CQI is most frequently called on to survey clients of behavioral health services to help the system or program improve the quality of its care[3]. Quantitative questions are designed to be actionable, and interviewers ask for comments when a respondent provides a negative response. In addition, CQI asks several open-ended questions to give overall context to the hard data. Demographic information is collected, and often used for comparative purposes. Reports are written that include recommendations. CQI staff meet with both provider staff and the funder (DMH, MBHP) to attempt to secure implementation of the recommendations. Thus, when CQI surveyed at several day programs a few years ago, some clients said that they had not been provided with clear mandate to call a specific crisis line if they were in crisis. In all cases, providers made improvements in response to CQI recommendations, as evidenced by follow-up CQI surveys.

CQI also leads qualitative evaluations of new and unique programs. In this case, CQI collaborates with consumers and other stakeholders to develop an interview guide, interviews clients shortly after they start the program and at intervals thereafter, and prepares the data for review, publication, or both. For example, in 2002, the Boston Medical Center obtained a SAMHSA grant to initiate and research a 8-bed Safe Haven shelter, which provides housing and services in a low-demand setting for people who are chronically homeless, actively substance abusing and have severe mental illness. CQI staff are members of project steering committee, and they are part of the research team, having helped to develop the research design. More specifically, CQI is leading the effort to learn about resident experiences, working with the evaluation committee to develop the interview guide, conduct interviews, code data and conduct data analysis.

CQI also conducts qualitative needs assessments, identifying consumer needs and desires, particularly with regard to service delivery and community supports. CQI reports not only on data collected, but offer recommendations for systems improvement. Recent examples of such reports include Voices of Youth in Transition: The Experience of Aging out of Public Mental Health Services in Massachusetts: Practice and Policy Implications, and DMH Clients and Employment in Western Massachusetts: The Consumer Perspective.

Action Focus

CQI conducts all of its research and evaluation with the goal of influencing policy and practice. CQI makes special efforts with its ongoing clients to relate their findings to action steps, and has met with some success. (Delman, 2004). When CQI discusses a project with potential collaborators, it is always with the intent of creating action from the data collected, including the targeting of specific audiences. (The Results section below contains some examples of the action focus of CQI's research.)

---

[3] Quality improvement interviews focus on a particular level of service, with interviewers using semi-structured surveys developed by CQI. CQI has developed and used surveys to interview clients of acute inpatient hospitals, day treatment programs, outpatient therapy/medication management services, Structured Outpatient Addiction Programs, state hospitals, Community Rehabilitation Services (CRS), DMH case management services, Program for Assertive Community Treatment (PACT) services and outpatient child/adolescent services

RESULTS

CQI survey research demonstrates a successful process of involving individuals with mental health disabilities in all aspects of research and evaluation, resulting in improved mental health practice and policy in Massachusetts. Below is table reporting CQI's survey research output over its first five years, followed by several examples of the impact of that output.

OUTPUTS AND IMPACT

(as of March, 2005)

Output	Impact
I. Quality Improvement Interviews[1]	
3000 People using MBHP 1000 People using DMH	-Stimulates respondents' critical thinking about recovery and support services. -Respondents appreciate the chance to express views to an objective and nonjudgmental person. -Collects significant data that is difficult to obtain. -Interviewers connect people with types of assistance (e.g., human rights officer, advocacy organization) that respondents were not aware of. -On rare occasions, interviewers have reported possible abuse to authorities.
II. Quality Improvement Reports	
218 Individual Programs	-Recommendations result in changes in provider policy and practice. -Providers adopt best practices identified by CQI. -MBHP or DMH takes decisive action when CQI notices a serious deficiency.
12 Aggregate Reports by Program Type	-Recommendations result in changes in industry policy and practice. -MBHP and DMH adopt professional training and education program to address areas of weakness. -CQI's publications educate public to advocate for systems improvements. -Results inform QI process and future research.

OUTPUTS AND IMPACT

Output	Impact
III. Qualitative Needs Assessment Reports (6 reports)	
Examples of Reports:	-Public awareness of issues is raised.
Vocational Assistance Needs of Western Massachusetts DMH Clients	-Reports impact the redesign of the service system in Massachusetts.
The Experience of Youth Aging Out of Public MH Services in Massachusetts	- DMH and MBHP take strategic and funding action to remediate problems and transform system.
The Better World Report: Key Areas of Systems Change Desired by DMH clients	-DMH and MBHP obtain guidance in redesigning Request for Proposals for specific types of services.
Quality of Life for MBHP members	-Consumer and family groups identify advocacy priorities.
IV. Qualitative Evaluation of New Programs	
Examples of Programs Evaluated:	-Articles and presentations contribute to literature.
Coordinated Family Focused Care: Family centered care for families with child with a serious emotional disorder.	-Service recipients appreciate the opportunity to influence their program by offering comments about its strengths and weaknesses.
Safe Haven Initiative: Transitional housing for people who are dually diagnosed with mental illness and chemical dependency, and formerly homeless.	-Aggregated information from interviews, integrated with other program data, is used to shape program development. -Reports help to insure that the program is responsive to the needs of the clients.
Real Choice: Self-directed care voucher program for people with disabilities and senior citizens.	

EXAMPLES OF IMPACT OF CQI SURVEY RESEARCH

Change in Provider Practice and Policy

Program for Assertive Treatment Team (PACT)

PACT[4] teams were initiated in Massachusetts in the last few years as an evidenced based practice- a team approach to working with people at risk for hospitalization in the community.

---

4 Program for Assertive Community Treatment, usually run by private vendors.

CQI conducted a series of qualitative interviews with clients who were considered least satisfied with the program, and CQI participated in team audits, sitting in on staff meetings where clients and case lists were discussed.

After several audits, CQI's analysis for the Department of Mental Health was that the team leader was perhaps the critical piece for the program's success, and that consumers often reported that the "approachability," or lack thereof, of that person was an important personal quality. We reviewed the team leader job descriptions being used, and found that they lacked a discussion of the necessary personal qualities that would make them approachable. Thus, CQI drafted a new job description and hiring guidelines for this program. These documents were accepted by DMH and passed on to providers, with strong encouragement to use them. As a result CQI's site recommendations and utilization of the new documents, several team leaders were removed for poor performance, and the quality of the teams improved.

POLICY CHANGES

Youth in Transition Needs Assessment

In 2000, CQI obtained a "consumer seed action grant" from Center for Health Care Strategies in order to develop a formal mechanism by which young adults with mental illness can influence state policies and practices related to the "aging out" process ("Young Adults in Transition Citizenship Project"). Two young adults were hired right away to help with survey design and raising awareness of the project in the community.

CQI then interviewed 24 young adults who had aged out of the adolescent mental health system in Massachusetts, then wrote the well-publicized report: Voices of Youth in Transition: The Experience of Aging Out of the Public Mental Health Service System in Massachusetts: Policy Implications and Recommendations.

Even before the project was completed, the two young adults were appointed co-chairs of the DMH Youth Development Committee. When they presented the results at key policy forums, they combined the hard data with their own personal stories of challenge and triumph. As a result, DMH began to fund both youth peer mentoring and youth advocacy training, and has begun to consider "transitional" case managers. CQI obtained funding for one of the young adults, who now works for DMH, to edit the booklet: "Recovery Stories Written by Inspiring Young Women," which DMH now uses as a training manual. The other young adult now works for M-POWER coordinating the peer mentoring project.

CHANGE IN INDUSTRY PRACTICE

Aggregate Reports

Utilizing its survey instrument statewide, CQI is able to write an aggregate report on the state of a provider industry, and permit individual providers to compare themselves to the norm and to each other. (These reports tend to have between 150 and 500 respondents.) CQI is also able to identify best practices so that providers and systems can learn from each other.

CQI is aware of community resources and has connected provider to them for quality improvement purposes.

For example, in writing a report on the responses of over 324 clients of 20 day programs, CQI learned that although day treatment clients were overall very satisfied with the care, some did not feel that their desire to work and otherwise be integrated back into society was supported. MBHP thus provided day programs with an opportunity to obtain consultation from the Boston University Center of Psychiatric Rehabilitation to help the programs become more recovery oriented. CQI also learned that in general clients did not know who the required Human Rights Officer was. MBHP sent out a quality alert with CQI's specific recommendations on this issue, and many programs changed their practices.

CONCLUSIONS

With the appropriate support, leadership, and collaboration, people with mental illness are able to lead survey research activities that promote health care best practices. Consumer leadership in policy and research promotes change since consumers tend have less stake in the current state of affair and in general recognize what their needs are and what might help them

It is important that the survey process be done with an action agenda in mind, which for CQI is not just accurate evaluation, but which promotes the best care practices and policies. Thus, it is important that this kind of survey research be a collaborative process, supported and embraced by other key stakeholders, such as government, providers, and other consumers.

A critical competent for success here is strong and savvy consumer direction, and purposeful hiring and supervision of staff. Building a mission driven business requires not only technical skill, but a political acumen. Ultimately, it is not simply strong consumer leadership that will lead to success, but also strong governmental leadership, which Massachusetts has offered. In addition, other stakeholders, such as providers and other consumer and family groups, have been supportive.

IMPLICATIONS

CQI's experience provides tangible evidence confirming that people within all disability groups have the capacity to direct and conduct survey research activities, with a likely result of improved and more responsive services. In fact, through a Real Choice CMS grant to Massachusetts, the state is working with people with a variety of disabilities to develop a self-directed voucher program, and CQI is working with the consumer and governmental steering committee to conduct qualitative surveys of people in the pilot program early on and then several months into the program. CQI's is thus bringing its methodology to other disability groups and sees survey research as another way for people can take greater charge of the systems and programs that serve them.

REFERENCES

Chaney, R. (2002, April), *The Value of Consumer Involvement in Medicaid Managed Care. Center for Health Care Strategies brief. Retrieved February 25, 2005 from the World Wide Web: http://www.chcs.org/usr_doc/consumer_involvement.pdf.*

Danley, K. S. and Ellison, M. L. (1997). *A handbook for participatory action researchers.* Boston, MA, Boston University, Center for Psychiatric Rehabilitation.

Deegan, P.E. (1993). Recovering our sense of value after being labeled mentally ill. *Psychosocial Nursing and Mental Health Services*, 31(4), 7-11.

Delman, J. (2004). Crossing the Mental Health Quality Chasm in Massachusetts. Retrieved February 25, 2005 from the World Wide Web: http://www.cqi-mass.org/quality-chasm.pdf.

Forquer, S., Sabin, J. (2002). Informed Purchasing Series Working Paper: What lies ahead. Center for Health Care Strategies. *Retrieved February 25, 2005 from the World Wide Web: http://www.chcs.org/usr_doc/bhforecasting.pdf.*

Gaventa, J. (1993). The powerful, the powerless, and the experts: Knowledge struggles in an information age. In P. Park, M. Brydon-Miller, B. Hall. and T. Jackson (Eds.) *Voices of Change: Participatory Research in the United States and Canada.* Westport, CT: Bergin, Garvey.

Harding, C.M., Brooks, G.W., Ashikaga, T., Strauss, J.S. and Breier, A. (1987a). The Vermont longitudinal study of persons with severe mental illness, I; methodology, study sample, and overall status 32 years later. *American Journal of Psychiatry,* 144(6) 718-726.

Holbrook, A.L., Green, M., and Krosnick, J. A. (2003). The Survey Response Process in Telephone and Face-to-Face Surveys: Differences in Respondent Satisficing and Social Desirability Response Bias. *Public Opinion Quarterly*, 67, 79-125.

Institute of Medicine. (2001). Committee on Quality Health Care in America, Crossing the Quality Chasm: *A New Health System for the 21st Century.* Washington, D.C., National Academy Press.

Israel, B. A., Schulz, A. J., Parker, E. A., Becker, A. B. , Allen, A. J., and Guzman, J. R. (2003). Critical Issues in Developing and Following Community Based Participatory Research Principles. In M. Minkler and N. Wallerstein (Eds.). *Community Based Participatory Research for Health* (pp 53-76) San Francisco: Jossey Bass.

Minkler, M., Blackwell, A. G., Thompson, M. and Tamir, H. (2003, August). Community-based Participatory Action Research: Implications for Public Health Funding. *Am J ofPublic Health*, 93(8), 1210-1213.

New Freedom Commission on Mental Health, Achieving the Promise: Transforming Mental Health Care: Final Report. (2003). Rockville, MD: *Department of Health and Human Services* Pub. No. SMA-03-3832.

Sabin, J., O'Brien, M. and Daniels, N. (2001). Managed care: strengthening the consumer voice in managed care: moving NCQA standards from rights to empowerment. *Psychiatric Services* 52, 1303-1305.

Sclove, R.E. (1997, Aug). Research by the people, for the people. Futures, 29(6) 541-549.

Simpson, E.L. and House, A.O. (2002). Involving users in the delivery of mental health services: systemic review. *British Medical Journal,* 325:1265-

Smith, L. W. (2000). The Rise of Consumer Satisfaction Teams. In Behavioral Outcomes and Guidelines Sourcebook (pp 384-395) New York: Faulkner and Gray.

Springett,J. (2003). Issues in Participatory Evaluation. In Minkler, M. and Wallerstein, N. (Eds.), *Community Based Participatory Research for Health* (pp 263-288) San Francisco: Jossey Bass.

Stoecker, R. (2002a, March). Thinking about CBR: Some questions as we begin. Keynote address presented at *"Best Practices in Undergraduate Community-Based Research: Challenges and Opportunities for the Research University"*, Ann Arbor, Michigan.

Strand, K., Marullo, S., Cutforth, N., Stoecker, R., and Donohue, P. (2003a). *Community-based research and higher education: Principles and practices.* San Francisco, CA: Jossey-Bass.

United States Public Health Service Office of the Surgeon General (1999). Mental Health: A Report of the Surgeon General. Rockville, MD: Department of Health and Human Services, *U.S Public Health Service.*

Viswanathan M., Ammerman A., Eng E., Gartlehner G., Lohr K.N., Griffith D., Rhodes S., Samuel-Hodge C., Maty S., Lux, L., Webb L., Sutton S.F., Swinson T., Jackman A. and Whitener L. Community-Based Participatory Research: Assessing the Evidence. Evidence Report/Technology Assessment No. 99 (Prepared by RTI—University of North Carolina Evidence-based Practice Center under Contract No. 290-02-0016). AHRQ Publication 04-E022-2. Rockville, MD: *Agency for Healthcare Research and Quality.* July 2004.

Wallerstein, N. and Duran, B. (2003). The Conceptual, Historical, and Practice Roots of Community Based Participatory Research and Related Participatory Traditions. In Minkler, M. and Wallerstein, N. (eds), *Community Based Participatory Research for Health* (pp 27-52) San Francisco: Jossey Bass.

In: Towards Best Practices for Surveying People..., Volume 1 ISBN 1-60021-195-X
Editors: Thilo Kroll, David Keer et al., pp. 89-103

Chapter 6

TRAINING TEMPORARILY ABLE-BODIED SURVEY INTERVIEWERS

Raymond E. Glazier

ABSTRACT

Even though one in five Americans has a disability, novice survey interviewers are often young people with little first-hand knowledge of different disabilities that they may encounter in the field. Therefore all in-person general population surveys, as well as those specifically targeting persons with disabilities, require interviewer training regarding, and sensitivity to various disabilities. This chapter summarizes an Interviewer Training Program developed by the author at Abt Associates Inc. An Interviewer Disability Training Manual, excerpted below, is custom-tailored to the specific survey's content, context, and particular population. Each trainee receives a bound copy of this manual, which is structured with reminder bullets and a quick reference Ten Commandments page, to read in advance of the training session.

The Americans with Disabilities Act of 1990 expanded the concept of disability to include:

- Persons with a history of disability or thought of by others as disabled.
- Persons with a history of psychiatric treatment.
- Excluded are persons with, for example, pyromania or pedophilia diagnoses, who might be thought likely to injure themselves or others.
- Persons in substance abuse recovery (but not active abusers).
- Protection is included for family members of persons with disabilities.
- Recent Supreme Court decisions have limited some of these protections.

In the one-day training session, the author, who has multiple severe disabilities (quadriplegia, speech impairment), first reviews the manual's content in a PowerPoint presentation. This is followed by a wide-ranging, free-wheeling discussion session in which no question is out of bounds.[1] Each trainee then draws a Chance Card that presents a problem interview situation, to which the trainee must role play and/or explain his/her response to the scenario.[2] Both the trainer and the other trainees critique the response of each trainee, providing suggestions, feedback, and positive input.

Abt interviewers trained with the first version of this manual successfully conducted 4,900 in-home interviews with persons with divers disabilities in an evaluation of Project NetWork, a Social Security Administration return-to-work experiment for SSI and SSDI beneficiaries. More recently the program was used to prepare site visitors, most of them able-bodied young women, to do in-home interviews with residents of subsidized housing projects for a Congressionally mandated HUD research project exploring residents' housing project size preferences. Respondents they successfully interviewed included adult males diagnosed with chronic mental illness and newly released prison inmates, as well as persons with developmental disabilities. The training program was found effective, in the view of the author's Abt Associates colleagues, in promoting interviewer confidence and capabilities, contributing to the accurate collection of difficult-to-obtain personal data. Field interviewers benefited from targeted training provided by a trainer with disabilities, in the view of their supervisors.

The interviewer training program abstracted here can readily be customized and replicated. The author is available to tailor the interviewer training program to any in-person survey and administer the training on-site for clients by consulting arrangement with Abt Associates Inc., 55 Wheeler Street, Cambridge, MA 02138. Dr. Glazier can be contacted by telephone at (617) 349-2481 / 617-489-1009 or via e-mail: Ray_Glazier@AbtAssoc.com or Ray_Glazier@post.Harvard.edu .

INTRODUCTION

Given that persons with disabilities will be found in any random sample of the general population (or most subsets thereof), it is important that interviewers be comfortable enough in interacting with persons with disabilities to be able to collect good data, and that respondents are comfortable enough to provide the same. Too often, our culture's emphasis on youth, good looks, and athleticism makes it seem that disabilities are "unusual" or "abnormal." Yet each and every one of us can be able-bodied only temporarily, and disability is simply a common aspect of the human condition. The popular culture's construction of disability as deviant can influence an interviewer to treat the respondent as an object of pity or even revulsion, as less than fully competent. It is vitally important for interviewers to *always* think of the respondent firstly *as a person*, and only secondarily as a person with a disability (or disabilities).

There is a wide range of disabilities that can occur across a person's life span:

- Physical disabilities like mobility impairments often come to mind first.

---

[1] The trainer was once asked if all quadriplegics have body odor. The person was generalizing from an experience with a quadriplegic boss who didn't shower often enough. Another query: "Do Deaf parents have Deaf offspring?" ("Sometimes, not always.")

[2] The Sample Situations included below in this chapter are actually Chance cards taken from a training for persons about to conduct in-home interviews with public housing residents with disabilities concerning their housing project size preferences, from a Congressionally mandated study Abt Associates conducted recently for HUD. The Commentaries on each are also drawn from this training. All materials in the training module are custom tailored to each particular survey project.

- But facial disfigurement is also a disability.
- Blindness or deafness may be complete or incomplete.
- Diseases like multiple sclerosis often wax and wane; they may be progressive.
- Conditions like diabetes may have multiple deleterious, disabling effects.
- Mental retardation occurs with different levels of severity.
- Mental health disabilities are less visible, but no less disabling, often intermittent and episodic.
- Similarly, substance abuse, even in recovery, affects many areas of life.
- Chronic illness, with or without chronic pain, can be very debilitating.

In situations where a friend, family member, or other caregiver must be involved in the interview as a proxy or "interpreter," the interviewer must keep in mind that the respondent is the focus of the interview and always direct attention to him or her. While there are many cases where a proxy might be able to answer the survey's questions more easily and quickly, data quality suffers when a third person is "second-guessing" the actual respondent. It is usually important to keep the reliance upon proxies to a *bare minimum,* using them only in cases where the interviewer simply cannot establish meaningful dialogue with the respondent. (The survey's sponsor ordinarily gives guidance on the matter of how liberally proxy respondents may be employed, and in what circumstances.)

The in-person survey interviewer must always keep in mind that he/she is a guest in the home of the respondent, and behave in the same manner, whether interviewing a person with or without any obvious disability. Interviewers may find themselves feeling more comfortable if they think of family or friends they know well who have disabilities. Chances are *one in five* that the interviewer's household itself has a person with a disability, since there are 53 million persons with disabilities in the United States, and the prevalence of disability is increasing (Fujiura, 2001).

Interviewers may not at first think of Aunt Bessie's thick glasses or Uncle Walter's cane as signs of a disability, but they are, in fact, indicative of disabilities. It is likely that *at some point* each and every one of us (if we live long enough) will have to deal with disability on a very personal basis. This is why disability activists sometimes speak of others as "temporarily able-bodied." It is even possible that some of the experiences interviewers encounter in survey research with persons with disabilities will provide them with valuable personal lessons for coping with disability (their own or a family member's) later in life.

Interviewing Pointers

In demographic terms, respondents with disabilities are statistically more likely to be of lower socioeconomic status, having lower educational achievement levels and lower than average incomes (Freedman, Martin, and Schoeni; 2004). Thus the demographic profile of potential respondents with disabilities does not mirror that of the general population, nor that of survey interviewers. Nevertheless, it is important that the interviewer strive to create an interviewing situation in which both parties are at ease. The tips presented in the following sections are intended to help eliminate any anxiety the interviewer may have.

In some cases the interviewer will have at least a rough idea of the respondent's disability. That information will make it fairly simple for the interviewer to look up the class of disability in the Interviewer Disability Training Manual, sections of which are abstracted below, and review both the generic and disability-specific tips and reminders before going to the interview. However, information of record about the respondent's disability may not square with his/her self-identification or the interviewer's assessment. Predisposing bias should be avoided by treating advance information with a certain degree of skepticism.

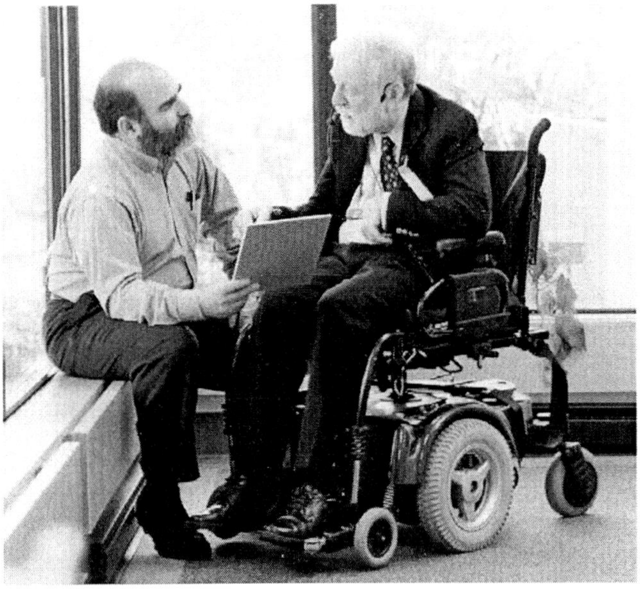

The interviewer should make sure that his/her disposition is positive and personable, but business-like. If the respondent's thoughts or attention wander from the substance of the interview, the interviewer needs to redirect the dialogue with a reminder of the specific reason for the visit. He/she must also be aware that the respondent may want to vocalize feelings that arise in reaction to particular questions. The interviewer should tolerate expressions of feelings, but be clear with the respondent when he/she does not answer the question and try to redirect the response by distinguishing between thoughts and feelings. (In most cases the interviewer is recording thoughts as answers, not feelings). Finally, the interviewer must be conscious that 'small talk' can be an important ice-breaker that personalizes the interview process. However, he/she should gently refrain from answering any personal questions the respondent might ask, by humorously reminding him or her that asking the questions is *the interviewer's job.*

Examples of Pointers

- When interviewing a wheelchair user, position yourself at his/her eye level.
- For a person with limited vision, find a well-lit area.

A few generic tips for in-person survey interviewers; some are generic to most interview situations, but take on even greater importance in the etiquette of interviews with persons with disabilities:

1) Always treat the person with a disability *as a person*; maintain eye contact with him or her.
2) *Do not* make assumptions about the person's mental or physical capacities that could be unwarranted and insulting.
3) Be careful of the words you use in connection with disabilities (see guidelines below), but do not become overly self-conscious about saying, for example, to a blind person, "I'm sure you see what I mean."
4) If another household member lets you in, be clear that it is the respondent you have come to see and that you and he or she will need as much privacy as can be managed.
5) If a third party is involved as proxy or interpreter, keep in mind who is the actual respondent and focus attention on him or her.
6) Try to free the room of other distracting influences (like a noisy TV or radio, active pets, playing children); suggest closing doors where it will help ensure privacy and/or cut down on background noise.
7) Allow the respondent to interrupt at any time with questions about the substance of the interview or comments about it. But try to resolve them quickly without breaking up the flow of the interview.
8) Repeat the question and response options as necessary, without taking on a condescending tone. Take notice of the respondent's demeanor and facial expressions; if he or she appears confused, offer to repeat the questions and response categories.

If you notice that a respondent appears extremely fatigued, offer to *temporarily discontinue* the interview (maybe state it as "taking a time-out"), given the understanding that it must be completed. (A few minutes' break and/or chat may suffice; at worst the interview may need to be completed later during a second visit.)

You may reserve some of these same rights for yourself, e.g., to ask for clarification if a response is not clear, or take a "time-out" if you need to collect your thoughts before going on.

Make it clear to the respondent that closed-ended questions must be answered with one of the response options offered, the one that "fits best," rather than allowing the person to give a different response and then try to "interpret it" into one of the response categories.

Be sure to give positive reinforcement to appropriate responses *without* appearing to reinforce the particular *content* of the response.

Allow yourself and the respondent the time you need to conduct a good interview. While it is not preferable to break off the interview until a later date, you may decide that this is the best way to acquire valid and reliable data from the respondent.

Language Pointers:

Several commonly used terms pertaining to disabilities are outdated, insensitive expressions, offensive to most individuals with disabilities, and in fact some respondents will not self-identify as "disabled," resenting a label they consider stigmatizing. Some of these common expressions are listed below, and recommended alternatives are provided. Note that acceptable usage is always in flux, as society's awareness of, and sensitivity to disability concerns continues to develop. Interviewers should avoid using any of the objectionable terms that are listed. As a general principle, we should always avoid using adjectives or participles as nouns (e.g. "the disabled"), which is disrespectful to the personhood of respondents (and others) with disabilities. It is always preferable to use "person first" language, e.g., to refer to "person(s) with x."

OBJECTIONABLE	PREFERRED
Afflicted with	Has a certain condition
Birth defect	Disabled since birth, born with
Cerebral-palsied	Has cerebral palsy
Cripple, crip	Walks with the aid of crutches, braces, etc.
Deaf mute	Deaf and speech impaired
Defective	Impaired, limited in respect
Disabled person,	Person with a disability, consumer (currently politically correct in most usage)
The disabled	Persons/people with disabilities
Deformed	Has a physical disability
Dummy	Pre-lingually Deaf, non-verbal
Elephant Man's disease	Neurofibromatosis
Emotionally disturbed	Person diagnosed with a psychiatric disability
Epileptic	Person with epilepsy, has a seizure disorder
Former mental patient	Mentally restored, psychiatric survivor
Handicapped	Has a disability
Handicapped accessible	Accessible to people with disabilities, fully accessible
Hearing impaired	Deaf or hard of hearing
Hunchbacked	Has a spinal curvature
Insane, deranged, deviant	Has a psychiatric disability
Lame	Walks with a limp, uses crutches
Midget, dwarf	Short-statured person, little person
Mongoloid idiot	Person with Downs syndrome
Normal	Non-disabled, able-bodied, temporarily able-bodied
Paralytic, arthritic	Person with paralysis, person with arthritis
Psycho	Person in recovery
Retard	Person with intellectual disability, or:
Retarded	Has an intellectual disability, is developmentally disabled
Spastic	Has seizures, muscular dystrophy, etc.

Suffers from	Has a specified condition, is a survivor of same
Wheelchair-bound	Wheelchair-active; uses a wheelchair / is a wheelchair user confined to a wheelchair

1. Cognitive Disabilities/Affective and Intellectual Disabilities

Mental retardation, better termed "intellectual disability," and mental illness, better termed "affective disability," are subjects often pointedly ignored. Yet these disabilities and other cognitive impairments like dyslexia and AD/HD (attention deficit / hyperactivity disorder) are fairly common and represent a sizeable segment of potential respondents who will likely be found in a general population sample. It is very important not to confuse these different disabilities and *never* to assume that the respondent cannot be approached on some level at which meaningful dialogue is possible, even if a third party must be involved.

Psychiatric Disability

Virtually all potential respondents who live with psychiatric disability control the condition through some combination of medication, professional therapy, and support groups. Many, if not most, forms of psychiatric disability are episodic in nature, and there may well be no effect whatsoever on the interview session. The interviewer may be privy to the presumed nature of the interviewee's disability from administrative records or from the nature of the specific survey and its sampling frame. But this information should be considered dubious (see above); the interviewer must try not to let this influence conduct of the interview. The interviewer should also remember that his/her mission is to respond respectfully to what may on occasion be emotional responses and accurately capture the respondent's perceptions.

Sample Situation: You were informed in advance that Sally is an intelligent, well educated person with two Ivy League degrees who has been diagnosed with schizophrenia. Sally is quite pleasant, offering you a cup of coffee when you come into her apartment. She tells you that she'd prefer <u>not</u> to live in this housing project with persons with disabilities, but has no choice about that just now because of her financial circumstances. At this point she wants to discontinue the interview, saying, " I just know the others are listening through the TV. That's why I never talk about private things in this room." What do you do?

Commentary: The important thing in this interview situation is to respond to Sally's feelings of the moment and seek a common ground that empowers her to decide whether or not to continue. A good reaction would be, "Well, then maybe you'd be more comfortable if we talk in another room. Where can we go to sit down and talk privately?"

Intellectual Disability

There are gradations of intellectual disability, and the interviewer should never assume in advance that a person is so cognitively impaired that communication cannot take place. It may be desirable, if feasible, to ascertain the respondent's recorded level of disability, but this information may be imprecise, inaccurate, and potentially misleading. In more severe cases, a family member or other third party may be able to help out with the interview. Only on rare occasions will a severe case of intellectual disability require use of a proxy for the interview. The interviewer must remember to keep the interview focused on the respondent rather than the third party, even when using a proxy. This means keeping eye contact with the respondent and acting as much as possible as if the third party were an invisible "translating machine." The interviewer needs to be alert to cues that the third party is "taking over" for the respondent, i.e., responding to questions before the respondent seems to recognize the meaning of the question and before he or she has reacted in any way. Here are some other pointers:

1) In presenting the survey, it may be possible to relate it to the individual's own experience and discuss the survey's purpose in terms of helping other people in the same situation in the future.
2) The interviewer should mentally evaluate the dialogue established with the first block of questions, so he/she can determine early on whether it is necessary to use a proxy for the interview.
3) Even if a proxy is required, it is necessary to have the actual respondent present for the duration of the interview, asking him/her to verify and validate responses from time to time and encouraging him/her to speak up if the proxy gets something wrong.
4) The interviewer must be aware that hypothetical examples might be taken very literally by the respondent.

Sample Situation: You are interviewing Ben, a 25-year-old man with moderate intellectual disability about his housing preferences. He is very shy and keeps looking to his father Harry, who is present to help with the interview. When you get to the question "What is the most important thing to you about where you live?" Harry says, without even looking to his son for a cue, "The most important thing for Ben is living near enough to us that his mother and I can look after him." How can you find out what *Ben* thinks? Commentary: While you do not want to come between father and son, the interviewer should probe for Ben's real feelings. What may be important for him might be friends (maybe a girlfriend) in the housing project where he lives. Or maybe he likes the fact that there is a good pizza parlor next door.

Learning Disability

There are a variety of disturbances in mental processes that can affect a person's verbal or mathematical abilities or the ability to listen, think, or speak. These may manifest themselves as difficulties with particular intellectual functions like reading, spelling, writing, or paying attention, but they may have little or no effect on the person's other mental abilities and functions. The interviewer must be alert for signs of fatigue and use short breaks as seems necessary.

Developmental Disabilities: *An Important Note*

People sometimes mistakenly assume that "developmental disability" is academic jargon for "mental retardation," or that the two terms are interchangeable. However, the term DD refers to onset *before age 22* of a mental *or* physical disability that may last indefinitely and that substantially limits three or more core areas of life activity from this list: mobility, learning, language (receptive and expressive), self care, self direction, independent living, and economic sufficiency.[3] Intellectual disability is only one *possible* (but not necessary) factor. Persons with developmental disabilities may constitute the largest single category in, for example, a survey of public housing residents with disabilities, and the interviewer should expect to find great variety in the severity and specific nature of these persons' impairments or disabling conditions. Recorded disabilities may tip off the interviewer as to what to expect of certain consumers he/she will be interviewing. But it is important that this advance information, which may in fact be incorrect or otherwise misleading, not predispose the interviewer to treat the respondent differently from another person one is meeting for the first time, for example, by approaching him or her as one might a child.

2. Sensory Disabilities

Hearing, sight, and speech disabilities, just like all others, vary in their degree. One must not assume that dark glasses, a white cane, or a guide dog necessarily imply complete loss of vision, any more than one would assume that a hearing aid indicates complete deafness. Interviews with respondents with sensory disabilities will, of necessity, take extra time, maybe even requiring a second visit to complete. In the following section we present some helpful hints for interviewers dealing with respondents who have disabilities involving sight, hearing, or speech.

Blindness/Limited Vision

Do remember that the person with legal blindness may have some residual sight.

1) Unless the person is totally blind, the interviewer should try to place him/herself under a light source, so that the respondent can have the best opportunity to visualize him or her.
2) If the respondent with blindness has a guide dog, the interviewer may ask permission to pet it briefly to establish friendliness, but *should not continue* to interact with it, as

---

[3] Source: http://www.cdc.gov/ncbddd/dd/default.htm, accessed 28 April 2005.

this may interfere with the dog's functioning to assist its owner. In no case should the interviewer pet the service animal without advance permission.

3) The interviewer must remember that papers and any other items he/she may have may not be entirely visible to the respondent. The respondent will benefit from a brief description of the materials and a running commentary on what one is doing. ("Now it will take me a minute to write down your response.")
4) When asking the questions and reading the response options (where provided), the interviewer should offer to repeat the question and response options on request, offering that option if the respondent looks confused or hesitant.

Deaf/Hard of Hearing

The term "hearing impairment" is actually no longer preferred usage; the current PC preference is for "Deaf" or "hard of hearing." One should be aware that persons born totally Deaf (or deafened before learning a vocal language) often (but not always) use American Sign Language (ASL) and consider themselves members of a Deaf (capital 'D') signing community that is a distinct and separate culture with its own language, etiquette, customs, etc.

The "culturally Deaf" person may consider ASL, *not English,* as his/her native language, and often distinguish other people who cannot hear as "**deafened**" (i.e., the past participle indicating having *acquired* deafness due to injury or illness after birth). There are also other manual communications methods: Pidgin Signed English (PSE) is distinct from ASL, as it uses English syntax and word order (unlike ASL); finger spelling is a manual way of representing each letter of the alphabet and takes considerable time to convey a message. Hispanic persons are likely to use other sign language systems that may vary by their country of origin. In some cases the respondent may be more comfortable utilizing a friend, family member, or caregiver who can interpret. When making arrangements for a hired sign language interpreter, the interviewer must be certain to match the needs of the respondent with the sign capabilities of the particular interpreter. Most cities of any size will have a Sign Language Interpreter Registry listed in the Yellow Pages.

It is important to be aware that the person who has been totally or almost totally Deaf for a long time, especially the person who was born so, may exhibit some degree of speech difficulty because of the absence (or severe limitation) of auditory feedback on how he or she sounds. The interviewer should be sure to review the section below on Speech Difficulty as well.

In discourse with a respondent who is Deaf or hard of hearing, the interviewer should be sure to maintain eye contact with the respondent, not the interpreter. It may be helpful to pretend that the interpreter is a robot, after the initial introductions and pleasantries. A trained professional interpreter will not feel excluded or offended if the interviewer acts as if he or she is not present, *except* for offering to break between sections of the survey instrument to give the interpreter a rest. The interviewer should be sure to sit in the light in full view of the interpreter so his/her face can be seen easily. In these interviews, enunciation is particularly important to the respondent who is Deaf or hard of hearing, as well as to the interpreter; one should *not* chew gum, smoke, or suck a lozenge during the interview. (Moustaches on male interviewers can also present problems to the lip reader.) It is important to pace oneself to speak slowly enough (with pauses as necessary) so that the interpreter can keep up. One should not ask the interpreter to clarify a respondent's answer, but ask the subject *through* the interpreter what was meant, if there is any uncertainty.

Some Deaf persons rely on a combination of residual hearing and lip reading to understand what is being said. In such situations, it is most important to be close to the subject and preferably under a light so one's face can be seen. (See generic cautions above about interfering factors.) The interviewer must suppress the all-too-natural tendency to shout, as excess volume can actually interfere with comprehensibility. Clear enunciation is usually more important, and it suffers when the voice is strained. This is especially true when one's voice is being amplified by hearing aids.

The person with adult onset hearing loss ("late deafened") may be reluctant to admit it, or to admit the degree of loss. Often such a person will have a spouse or other family member sitting alongside him or her, relaying the other person's conversation into the "better ear" in something like a stage whisper. As in other third party situations (see above), the interviewer must avoid the tendency to ask the interpreter to clarify or explain an unclear answer. The lay interpreter (family member, friend, or neighbor) can be more problematic as an interpreter because he or she may fully expect to participate in the substance of the dialogue.

A recap of some specific tips for the interview of a person who is Deaf or hard of hearing:

1) Eliminate any background noise by asking that TV or radio be turned off and doors shut.
2) Position oneself nearby and in the light for optimum audibility *and* visibility.
3) Speak distinctly, with clear (but not grotesquely exaggerated) lip movements. Do not raise one's voice unnecessarily.
4) *Do not* compromise the quality of the interview and the data being collected by trying to oversimplify questions in a misguided effort to make them more intelligible.
5) *Do keep in mind* that the person's hearing loss does not affect his / her mental acuity.
6) Maintain interview focus on the respondent and not any third party interpreter.
7) Do not be afraid to repeat a question or ask for clarification of an answer.

Deaf *and* Blind

An interview with the rare person who is both totally blind and Deaf might seem like a significant challenge. But the interviewer should realize, and arrange in advance that in such an interview his/her words will need to be communicated by a special sign language interpreter who will "finger spell" into the respondent's hand. This is an arduous and time-consuming process, but there will be rewards to seeing the subject "come to life," rapidly signing replies to the questions posed. The interpreter will then vocalize the meaning of the signed responses.

Speech Difficulty

The speech difficulty of the pre-lingually or long-term Deaf person has been noted above. Stuttering is another common speech difficulty with which the interviewer needs to be prepared to deal. The person who stutters is more likely to exhibit difficulty in interacting with a stranger (which, of course, the interviewer will be). He or she cannot control the problem, and the interviewer needs to be patient; trying not to rush the person, which will only contribute to the difficulty. It is also important for the interviewer to avoid the all-too-natural tendency to try to complete the person's sentence for him or her because the interviewer feels foolish waiting for the stutter to stop. When the stutter occurs at the end of the subject's sentence, the interviewer should be careful *not* to try to finish the respondent's sentence or talk over him or her by jumping ahead to the next question on the assumption that the respondent has nothing to add.

Other conditions that may interfere with the interviewer's understanding of the respondent's speech include: stroke, which may affect the mechanics of vocalization *or* vocabulary and use of words as symbols, paralysis (as in some traumatic brain injuries) of soft palate, lips, and/or tongue; and injury to, disease of, or surgical removal of the voice box. For example, the person who has had a laryngectomy (surgical removal of the voice box) sometimes speaks using *inhaled* rather than exhaled air, with or without the aid of a device inserted into the windpipe. One may experience some difficulty in getting accustomed to the phraseology dictated by this or other conditions limiting the person's air supply, as, for example, with the person whose breathing is assisted by a portable ventilator (Christopher Reeve style). Often the portable ventilator operates from the batteries of the person's electric wheelchair, with a large, ribbed transparent plastic tube carrying the air from the ventilator's backpack around to the front of the neck and directly into the windpipe.

A recap of some useful tips for interviewers interacting with a person with a speech difficulty include:

1) Don't try to rush the interview; place yourself where you can see and hear the respondent best.
2) Carefully avoid the tendency (all too human, but nonsensical) to speak more distinctly and loudly yourself, as if that would improve the respondent's vocalization.
3) Do not compromise the interview data by giving short shrift to difficult or open-ended questions, or by rephrasing questions too simplistically.
4) As mentioned earlier regarding deafness, remember that a speech disability does not affect mental acuity.
5) **Above all**, do not pretend you understand the response if you really do not. This kind of well intentioned bluff can result in an incorrect record of the response. And it can prove embarrassing later on in the interview when you might say something that will reveal your misunderstanding. Feel free to say something like, "This information is so important that I want to be sure I understood that. Could you please say it again, perhaps in a slightly different way?"

Tourette's Disease/Syndrome

This is a rare congenital disorder in which the person has nervous tics, involuntary movements, or inappropriate vocalizations over which he/she has no control. These tics may include any or all of the following: facial twitches or grimaces, sudden jabbing of a fist or kicking, involuntarily repeating a word or phrase just spoken by someone else, or involuntarily, often suddenly and explosively, uttering vulgar, obscene, or otherwise inappropriate words. This condition can cause great distress for an intelligent, sensitive person who cannot control these unwanted movements and/or vocal outbursts and be situationally problematic for the interviewer. It is important to realize that the movements and utterances, which may seem menacing, cannot be controlled by the subject any more than can stuttering. In fact, both difficulties can be aggravated and triggered by efforts to contain them or any feeling of being rushed.

The interviewer will probably know in advance of this disability, should he/she encounter it. The person who has lived with Tourette's knows that it is best to forewarn new contacts. When advised of this situation, the interviewer should ask how best he/she can help. In some cases the individual, who is otherwise cogent and very well spoken, will be free of involuntary vocalizations while speaking in answer to a question, but will experience them while trying to listen quietly to the interviewer. The interviewer can be helpful by ignoring the outbursts and focusing on the actual answers, not becoming flustered if his/her words are repeated involuntarily.

3. Mobility Disabilities

Mobility disabilities may result from paralysis or actual absence of limb dating from birth or acquired through illness or injury. Mobility devices used by these persons to get around and about may include: cane, walker, crutches, braces, prostheses (artificial limbs), or wheelchair (manual, electric, three-wheel "scooter"). Persons with severe mobility impairments, especially those persons who are quadriplegic (paralyzed to some degree in all four limbs), may need personal assistance services from a third party to function in the home setting. This helper person (often called a Personal Assistant, a PA, or a "PCA" for the now outdated term "personal care attendant") may answer the door and admit the interviewer. Usually the only reason for this person to remain in the room for the interview is *if the respondent or the interviewer feels more comfortable* having him/her at hand. All of the cautions about third parties (see above) apply; this person's role is that of facilitator or enabler, not proxy.

Sample Situation: You are interviewing Betty, a young woman with developmental disability who uses a wheelchair. She has told her personal assistant (PA) that he can go out for a smoke, so you can conduct the interview in private in her quarters. Things are going well despite Betty's moderate speech impairment, when suddenly her arms and legs begin to spasm in what appears to be a seizure, and her cup of coffee spills. What should you do?

Commentary: The important thing is to call the PA back into the room right away; he knows how to handle this. An all-to-human reaction is to worry about the spilled coffee, unless it is hot enough to burn Betty. *Do not* try to force something in her mouth to "prevent her swallowing her tongue" (a common mistaken notion).

The interviewer must, as with other physical disabilities, guard against assuming a connection between impairment of bodily functions and a limitation of mental faculties. He/she should be sure to discourage unnecessary presence of third parties, as this may compromise the confidentiality of the interview, and be careful not to address questions to any third party present. It is important for the interviewer to maintain eye contact with the respondent, treat him/her as the person one has come to see, and from whom one fully expects to get valuable information. At the same time, the interviewer should avoid voyeuristic staring or personal (not on the schedule) questions about the exact nature and origin of the disability, related difficulties, lifestyle implications, or particular causal circumstances. There is an all-too-human tendency to assume too great a degree of intimacy with a person who is in some way perceived as being in a "down position" relative to oneself. Asking what caused the disability, or when and how it occurred could be perceived as voyeurism.

With regard to the interviewee's wheelchair or other mobility device, the interviewer must not lean on it or try to push it, unless very specifically asked to do so. Otherwise one is invading that person's body space, of which the mobility device is an integral part. When addressing the person using a wheelchair or scooter, the interviewer should position him/herself near that person's eye level: In a brief encounter, one might hunker down; but for an extended conversation or for the interview itself, it will be more comfortable to pull up a chair and sit facing the person. The interviewer may offer assistance (for example, with a dropped article) as seems appropriate. But the interviewers should not jump up to do something without asking first to make sure the help is welcome. And he or she should not feel rebuffed or insulted if the offer is declined.

A few important reminders for interviewers:

1. Assume an active mind with which one can interact, disregarding the body.
2. Don't stare at bodily anomalies, disfigurements, missing limbs, unusual equipment.
3. Do not ask the respondent's personal assistant (PA) to assist you.
4. Do not speak over the wheelchair user's head to a third person as if he/she were the proxy.
5. One may offer help by asking, "May I help you?" If the respondent answers affirmatively, then ask, "How?" In this way, one can avoid doing something the person would prefer to do him/herself. This applies to pushing wheelchairs, pulling out table or chairs, and other types of personal assistance.

General

Many persons with disabilities have experienced negative interactions with strangers; they will appreciate being treated with common courtesy and respect. In most situations, particularly those in which communication is problematic, the interviewer should encourage the respondent to express his or her thoughts completely, accepting a longer answer than the one or two words recording the response. As the survey interviewing progresses and the interviewer conducts more and more interviews, he/she will become more comfortable and confident about surveying people with disabilities. It is important to realize that assistance is always available from a field supervisor. The experience of interviewing persons with disabilities will most likely be educational, enjoyable, and awareness-raising for the survey professional.

REFERENCES

Freedman, Vicki A., Linda C. Martin, and Robert F. Schoeni (2004). Disability in America. *Population Bulletin*, Vol. 59, No. 3

Fujiura, Glenn T. (2001). Emerging Trends in Disability. *Population Today*, August/September 2001.

AUTHOR NOTE

Raymond E. Glazier is founder and Director of the Abt Associates Center for the Advancement of Rehabilitation and Disability Services. His decades of research in this field, including numerous consumer surveys, have resulted in many publications on a broad range of disability issues in education, employment, health care, legal rights, housing, and vocational rehabilitation. Much of Dr. Glazier's current work focuses on the intersection of employment and health care coverage for persons with all types of disabilities, with particular interest in consumer direction of personal assistance services (PAS). He is a Harvard-trained sociologist who holds the

Ph.D. in social policy from Brandeis University's Heller School for Social Policy and Management.

In: Towards Best Practices for Surveying People..., Volume 1 ISBN 1-60021-195-X
Editors: Thilo Kroll, David Keer et al., pp. 105-125

Chapter 7

INCLUSION OF PEOPLE WITH DISABILITIES IN THE NHIS AND NHIS-D: NON-RESPONSE, PROXY RESPONSE, AND ASSISTED RESPONSE

H. Stephen Kaye
Disability Statistics Center and Center for Personal Assistance Services
University of California, San Francisco

ABSTRACT

Proxy response, which occurs when a person responds to a survey on behalf of another family member, is often used to obtain information about people who cannot respond for themselves, do not wish to respond, or are not available to do so. Although proxy response is generally better than non-response, it can introduce bias, especially when questions are personal, sensitive, or highly subjective. This chapter evaluates two efforts by the U.S. National Center for Health Statistics to increase self-response to surveys. In Phase II of the National Health Interview Survey on Disability, a substantial increase in self-response was achieved among a broad sample of people with disabilities. However, people with severe physical, cognitive, or speech disabilities were very likely to be responded for by proxy. Non-response to the survey was generally quite low. In contrast, introduction of a self-response only rule to the Sample Adult section of the National Health Interview Survey resulted in high non-response overall, in particular for people with mobility or cognitive impairments. Subsequent relaxation of the rule to allow proxy response in certain cases greatly reduced non-response, but at the cost of abandoning the goal of obtaining self-responses from all types of respondents, including those with severe disabilities. Assisted response, in which the person responds with help from a family member or caregiver, is proposed as a middle ground between self- and proxy response for people who have difficulty answering survey questions.

INTRODUCTION

Federal survey procedures often allow one adult to answer questions on behalf of an entire family or household. When this *family respondent* (or *household respondent*) supplies information about other members of the household, those other members are said to have responded *by proxy*. Proxy response is permitted partly because it saves money by reducing the need for repeated contacts with each household. It also reduces both non-response and sampling bias by assuring collection of data on all household members, rather than just those people who are at home when contact attempts are made.

Even for surveys in which self-response is sought for all adult participants, proxy response is sometimes allowed when a person is unavailable, unwilling, or deemed unable to respond. The "unable" category includes people with disabilities who may not have been offered the accommodations they would need to respond for themselves, such as a sign language interpreter, an interview conducted in stages to allow rest periods, or an interview conducted in an alternative mode—in person rather than over the phone, or by phone rather than on paper. In the absence of such accommodations, many people with disabilities are prevented from answering questions for themselves; some, who may not live with family members who can respond for them, are excluded from the data collection entirely.

For objective, straightforward questions whose answers are well known by the other adults in the household (for example, basic demographic information or employment status), proxy responses might generally yield valid data (see, e.g., Hendershot, 2003), but when the questions are more subjective or personal in nature, validity of proxy answers is more likely to be suspect (Andresen, Vahle, and Lollar, 2001; Dorman, Waddell, Slattery, Dennis, and Sandercock, 1997; Perry and Felce, 2002; Rothman, Hedrick, Bulcroft, Hickam, and Rubenstein, 1991; Stancliffe, 1999; Tamim, McCusker, and Dendukuri, 2002; Todorov and Kirchner, 2000). Questions designed to identify people with disabilities generally have a least some degree of subjectivity—for example, whether the person regards himself or herself as able to work, the degree of difficulty the person has climbing a flight of stairs, or the extent to which a person's mental health limits his or her daily activities. The last example, and the general task of identifying people with mental health disabilities, also involves questions of a personal nature, the true answers to which may not be known by the family respondent.

Disability and health surveys often include numerous personal, subjective questions, accurate responses to which are crucial for understanding the status of people with disabilities and comparing it to that of people without disabilities. These may include questions on quality of services received, experiences of perceived discrimination, attitudes toward and perception of disability status, and satisfaction with social life. Proxy responses to such measures might be of dubious value. Responses to questions on adequacy of help received with activities of daily living (ADL), for example, might be suspect when supplied by the family member who provides that help (LaPlante, Kaye, Kang, and Harrington, 2004).

For two Federal surveys with substantial disability content, data collection procedures were developed to increase self-response and presumably improve the validity of the data collected. In one such effort, a survey of people with disabilities known as Phase II of the National Health Interview Survey on Disability (NHIS-D), interviewers were specially trained in interacting with people with disabilities and were instructed to obtain self-responses whenever possible. The second effort involves the annual general population survey known as the National Health Interview Survey (NHIS). In 1997, following a major redesign of the survey, much of the content was moved into a module to be administered to only one randomly selected adult per household, and proxy responses to this module were initially not permitted, and later permitted only in extreme circumstances.

In this chapter, we evaluate the extent to which these changes in survey procedures have been effective in ensuring overall participation, and in particular self-representation, of people with disabilities in these surveys.

THE NATIONAL HEALTH INTERVIEW SURVEY ON DISABILITY, 1994–97

The National Health Interview Survey is a nationally representative household survey conducted annually by the Census Bureau for the National Center for Health Statistics (NCHS), part of the Centers for Disease Control and Prevention. Respondents to the 1994 and 1995 NHIS also took part in two supplemental surveys, known collectively as the National Health Interview Survey on Disability. Developed and funded by a consortium of federal agencies and the Robert Wood Johnson Foundation, the NHIS-D was designed to gather detailed data on the U.S. community-resident population with disabilities (National Center for Health Statistics, 1998). In Phase I of the NHIS-D, which was administered at the same time as the NHIS core, 202,560 persons were screened for any indication of disability, using an extensive set of criteria including functional limitation, specific disabling diagnoses, perception of disability, and use of disability-related services. Interviews were generally conducted in person with adult members of the sample family who were at home at the time of the interview.

A complex set of eligibility criteria was used to identify a sample of persons who fell within one or more of several conceptual or programmatic definitions of disability; these persons were to be interviewed again at a later date as part of the second phase of the NHIS-D. The Phase II questionnaire, also known as the Disability Followback Survey, contained detailed questions on employment, use of services, benefits, transportation, personal assistance needs, housing characteristics, environmental barriers, and participation in social activities. Data collection began in September 1994 and concluded in April 1997, with interviews taking place between 7 and 26 months following the Phase I interview. The Phase II sample numbers 32,788 persons, most of whom were interviewed in person, with the remainder interviewed by telephone.

In conducting Phase II of the NHIS-D, NCHS and the Census Bureau made a special effort to obtain self-responses for as many as possible of the people identified as having disabilities in Phase I. Survey takers (known as "field representatives") were instructed to go to extra effort to speak directly with the eligible person with a disability, and they were given special training in methods of interacting with people with disabilities, in order to obtain complete and accurate self-responses (Cynamon, 1994; U.S. Bureau of the Census, 1993). Despite the inclusion of substantial disability content in the NHIS since its inception, this was the first time that field representatives had been instructed in procedures for interviewing people with disabilities who might experience communication or other barriers to participation.

RESPONSE TO PHASE I

For the NHIS core, as well as for Phase I of the NHIS-D, the survey's usual interview procedures were followed, and all adult family members who were present at the time of the interview were invited to participate in the interview. Among households responding to the survey, 61.9 percent of adults responded to the Phase I questionnaire for themselves, in whole or in part, meaning that they were present for at least part of the interview. This rate compares favorably with surveys that routinely accept information from the family respondent alone; the monthly Current Population Survey, for example, achieves only a 53.8 percent self-response rate for its labor force questions.[1]

People with disabilities were actually more likely to respond to Phase I for themselves than people without disabilities. As shown in Figure 1, 70.2 percent of adults who were limited in activity self-responded, compared to 59.9 percent of those not limited in activity. Using the more complex set of criteria for identifying adults with disabilities who would be eligible to be interviewed in Phase II, 72.1 percent of eligible adults responded for themselves, compared to 59.2 percent of adults who were ineligible for Phase II, and therefore presumably had no indication of disability. These differences can be explained by the greater proportion of people with disabilities who live alone, and therefore cannot normally be responded for by proxy, and the greater proportion who are not working, and therefore more likely to be at home when the interviewer arrives or calls, When the sample is restricted to people not living alone and not employed, the self-response rates are equal for people with and without disabilities.

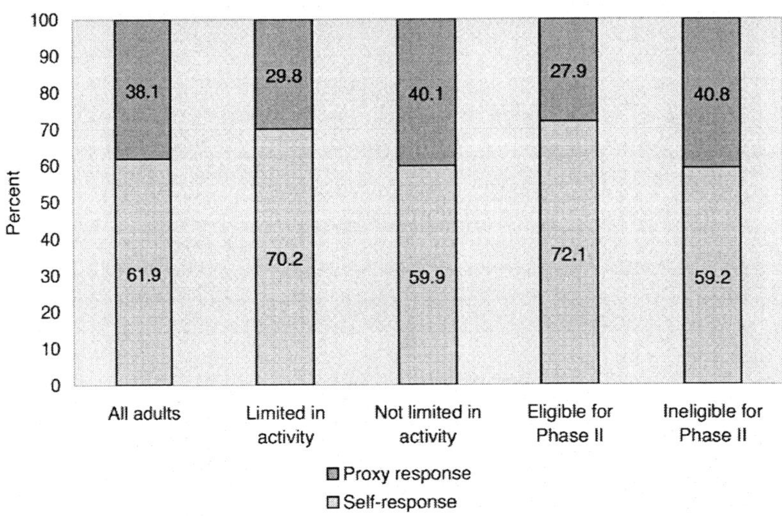

Figure 1. Type of response to NHIS-D Phase I among adults

RESPONSE TO PHASE II

Turning to Phase II of the NHIS-D, we find that NCHS succeeded in their efforts to increase self-response. Among people who participated in both parts of the survey—meaning that they self- or proxy responded to Phase I, were found eligible for Phase II based on some indication of disability, and self- or proxy responded to Phase II—the rate of self-response is substantially greater in the second phase. As shown in Figure 2, the self-response rate was 82.3 percent among Phase II respondents, a 10 percentage-point increase over the 72.4 percent of the same respondents who reported for themselves in Phase I (slightly greater than the 72.1 percent for all people eligible for Phase II, not all of whom were interviewed; survey non-response will be discussed later in this chapter).

For people who were not able to respond entirely by themselves, Phase II allowed the possibility of responding with the help of another person. The rate of *assisted response*, as distinct from the case of proxy response in which the person of interest does not participate, is 4.8 percent. Adding this group to the 82.3 percent who responded entirely by themselves, we obtain an impressive total of 87.1 percent of Phase II respondents reported for themselves, with or without assistance, while the remaining 12.9 percent were spoken for entirely by someone else.

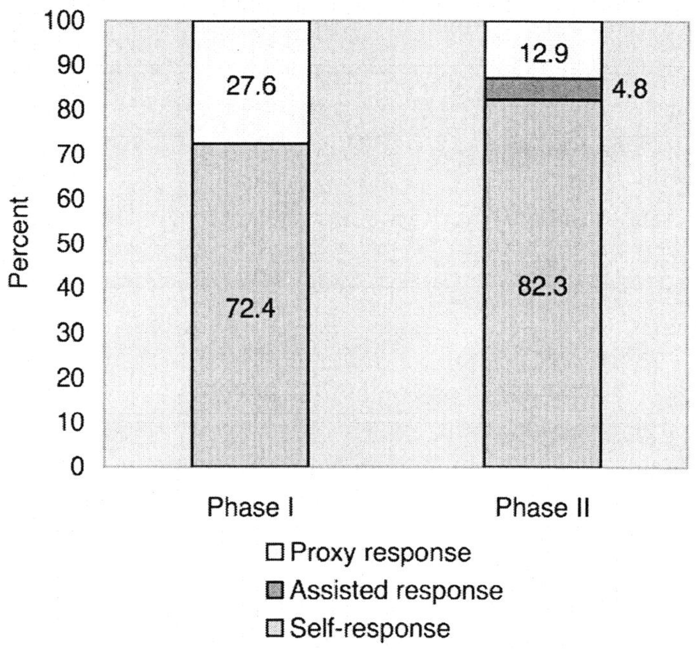

Figure 2. Type of response to Phase I and II among adult responsents to NHIS-D Phase II

The rate of proxy response is not uniform across disability subpopulations, but instead generally increases with disability severity and in the presence of certain types of disabilities. One severity measure is the number of activities of daily living that a person gets help with.

[1] Based on author's tabulation of data from adult respondents to the September 2004 Current Population Survey.

Using the basic set of five ADLs (bathing, dressing, eating, transferring, and toileting), we find a steadily increasing share of proxy response as the number of ADLs increases (Figure 3). People who get no ADL help had a proxy rate of only 11.4 percent, nearly doubling to 22.3 percent for one ADL (a highly statistically significant increase[2]) and further increasing to between 34 and 40 percent for people getting help with between 2 and 4 ADLs. For those getting help in all five ADLs, the proxy rate is 63.6 percent—nearly two-thirds of respondents (again, the increase is highly statistically significant).

Rates of assisted response are also greater for people getting ADL help, doubling from 4.4 percent for those not getting help to 8.9 percent for those getting help in one ADL (the difference is highly statistically significant). For people getting help with more than one ADL, the average is 11.3 percent assisted response (not a significant difference compared to one ADL).

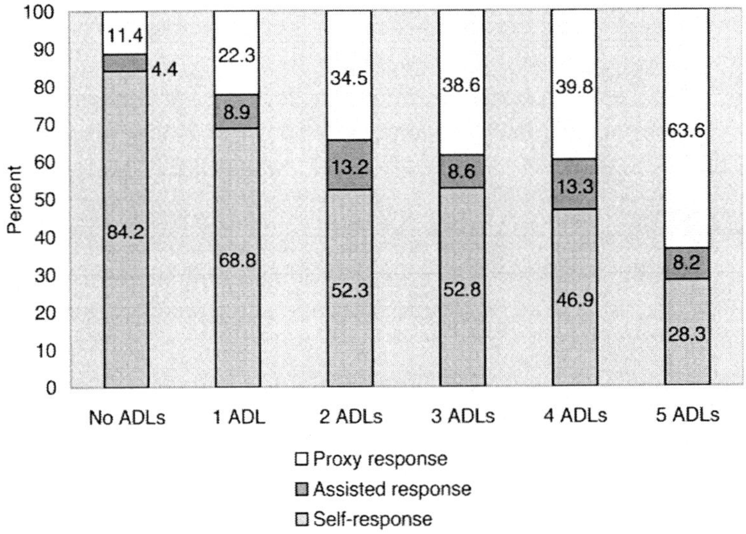

Figure 3. Type of response to NHIS-D Phase II, by number of ADLs

RESPONSE BY IMPAIRMENT TYPE

People receive help with ADLs generally because of mobility or cognitive limitations, or often both. Cognitive impairments would seem particularly relevant to survey response. As shown in Figure 4, people with severe cognitive limitations (regardless of ADL status) have very high rates of proxy response: 76.9 percent for people with Alzheimer's and 69.1 percent for people with mental retardation. People with learning disabilities, a milder form of cognitive impairment, also have a significantly higher rate of proxy response than those without cognitive limitations, 19.9 percent versus 11.2 percent.

---

2 Fisher's exact test is used to evaluate the statistical significance of these comparisons; because the tabulations are of respondents (unweighted) rather than the population represented (weighted), the complex survey design is not taken into account in these estimates.

Assisted response is more than twice as likely for people with severe cognitive limitations as for those without cognitive limitations (10.7 percent for Alzheimer's and 9.7 percent for mental retardation, significantly above the 4.7 percent for no cognitive limitation). Those enabled with assistance to answer questions for themselves nonetheless represent a small fraction of all respondents with these cognitive limitations.

Among people with mobility impairments (Figure 5), only those with the most severe level of difficulty have high rates of proxy response. Some 41.0 percent of this group, people needing and receiving assistance getting around the house[3], are responded for by proxy. For those with lesser levels of mobility limitation, the proxy response rate is 14.7 percent, compared to 11.8 percent for those without mobility limitations.

Assisted response is also significantly greater for those with severe mobility impairments, at 10.8 percent, compared to 7.4 percent for those with other mobility impairments and 4.2 percent for those without mobility impairments.

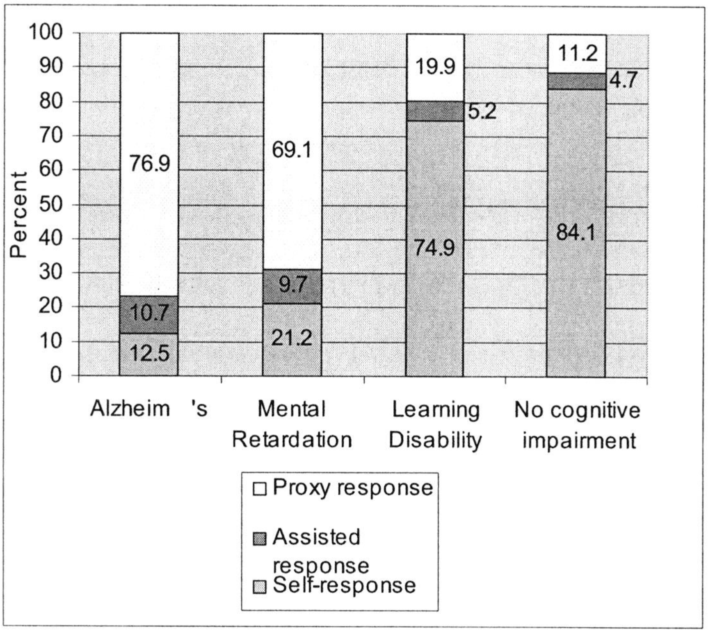

Figure 4. Type of response to NHIS-D PhaseII, by cognitive impairment

Another group with high rates of proxy response is people with speech impairments. As shown in Figure 6, more than half (56.5 percent) of people with severe speech impairments (defined as those whose speech is reported as difficult to understand by family members) responded by proxy, as did just under half (47.7 percent) of those with moderate speech impairments (speech reported as difficult to understand by strangers but not family members). The group with a lesser degree of impairment has a significantly higher rate of assisted response, at 11.0 percent, than the more severe and unimpaired groups, at 4.8 and 4.7 percent, respectively.

[3] This measure is treated as an ADL in the survey but not in this analysis.

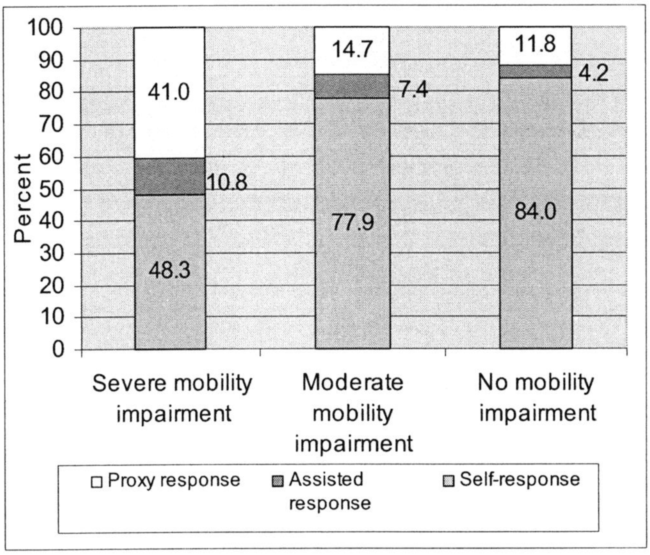

Figure 5. Type of response to NHIS-D PhaseII, by mobility impairment

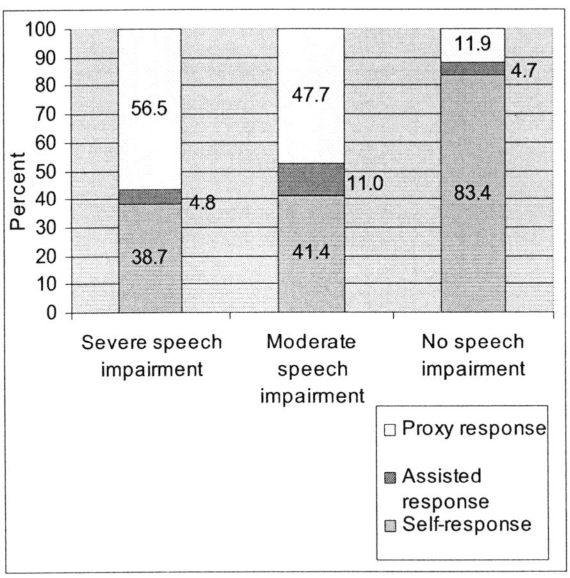

Figure 6. Type of response to NHIS-D PhaseII, by speech impairment

People with severe sensory impairments also have relatively high rates of proxy response, but at nothing like the levels for people with speech impairments. One-quarter (25.0 percent) of deaf people and about one-sixth (17.1 percent) of blind people were spoken for by someone else (Figure 7). People with moderate sensory impairments had only slightly higher rates of proxy response than people without such impairments.

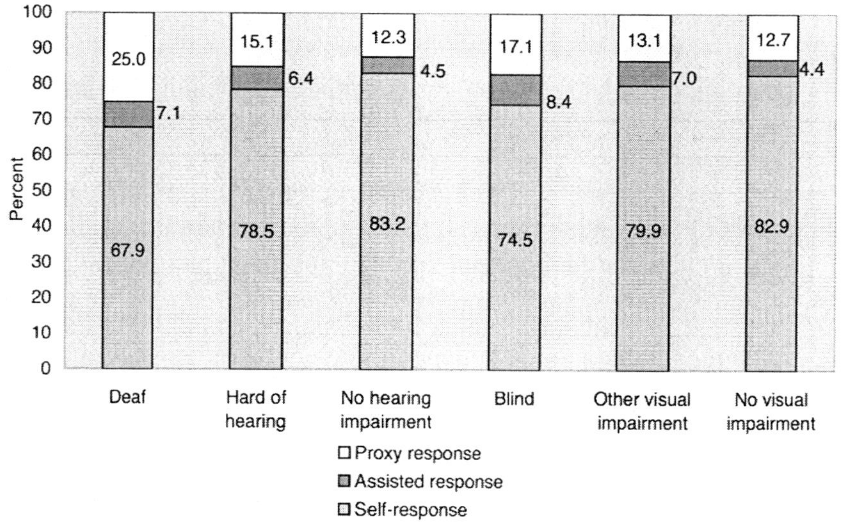

Figure 7. Type of response to NHIS-D PhaseII, by sensory impairment

For people with moderate and severe levels of visual or hearing impairments, rates of assisted response are significantly higher than for those without sensory impairments. These rates range from 6.4 to 8.4 percent, compared to about 4.5 percent for people with no sensory impairments.

A final group is people with mental health disabilities (Figure 8). People with psychoses (schizophrenia or some other paranoid or delusional disorder) were spoken for by proxy in 23.4 percent of cases, about twice the rate (11.9 percent) for people with no mental health disability. People with other mental health disabilities (reported as having mental health symptoms that interfere with daily activities) had a 20.8 percent proxy response rate.

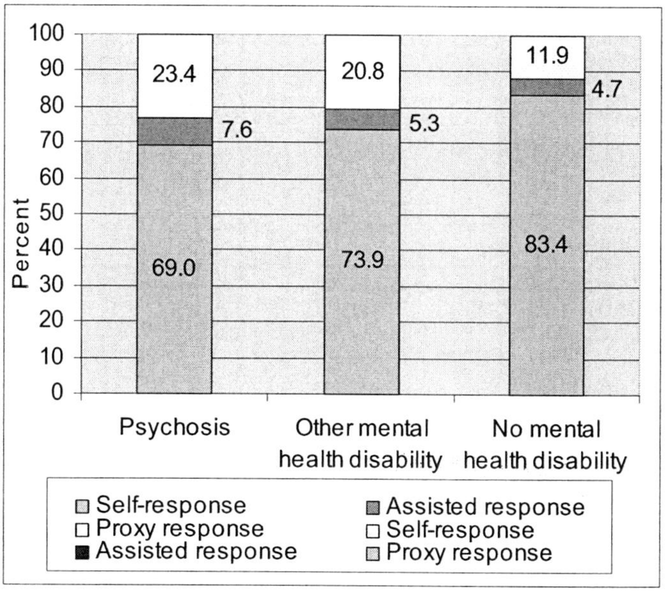

Figure 8. Type of response to NHIS-D PhaseII, by mental health disability

Modeling Phase II Response

One complication in interpreting the rates of proxy and assisted response is that many people have multiple causes of disability. Because some types of disability often occur alongside other types (for example, people who experience aging-related mobility limitations also often experience hearing loss or cognitive impairments), it is difficult to know whether to attribute lack of self-response to one source versus another. Efforts to improve self-response, however, require an understanding of exactly which barriers typically prevent people from self-responding.

A further complication is that there are reasons for proxy response that are unrelated to disability. People may be too busy to participate, may be away for an extended period of time, or may simply prefer not to respond. Such factors are likely to vary according to a person's age, gender, and socioeconomic circumstances. In the case of assisted response, a person may simply rely on another household member to have a better recollection of health-related episodes and services received.

By constructing separate models of proxy and assisted response as functions of impairments and other factors, we can try to isolate the effect of each type of impairment on the type of response. In separate logistic regressions of the likelihood of proxy or assisted response, we control for age (and age^2), sex (and an age-sex interaction), and educational attainment (using seven dummy variables indicating educational attainment above or below high school graduation). Dummy variables for each of the impairments shown in Figures 4 through 8 are also included. Based on the regression coefficients obtained in the models, we estimate the rate of proxy or assisted response for a person with each type of impairment, controlling for personal factors and any other impairments the person might have.

Shown in Figure 9 are the rates of proxy and assisted response obtained from the models. Severe cognitive impairments are associated with by far the highest proxy rates, between five and six times the proxy rate of the residual category of those without any of the listed impairments. Also quite high are rates for people with speech impairments and those with severe mobility impairments—those needing assistance to get around the house.

Deaf people and people with severe mental health disabilities, associated with psychoses like schizophrenia, also have proxy response rates substantially greater than for the residual group. People with lesser cognitive or mental health disabilities have slightly higher proxy rates than the residual group, when personal factors and other impairments are controlled for.

The highest levels of assisted response are among people with psychoses, whose rate is just over twice that of the residual group. Other groups with relatively high rates of response with assistance are those with severe mobility impairments, mental retardation, learning disabilities, and blindness. The lowest rates—less than half that of the residual group—are for people with speech impairments severe enough that their family members have trouble understanding them.

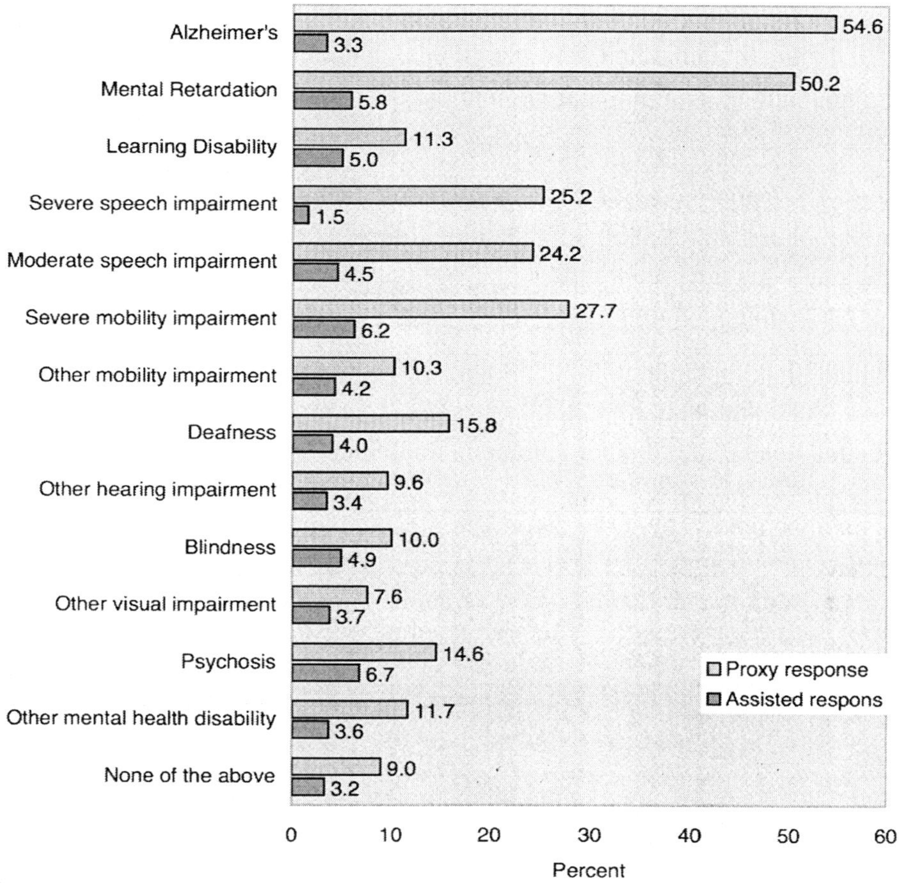

Figure 9. Rate of proxy and assisted response to Phase II of the NHIS-D, by impairment type, controlling for demographics and other impairments

PHASE II NON-RESPONSE

So far we have focused on adults who responded to Phase II of the NHIS-D, either answering for themselves, with or without assistance, or by proxy. Respondents comprise 89 percent of the adults who were deemed eligible for the survey, based on information collected in Phase I. The Phase II non-response rate of 11.0 percent[4] is remarkably low for a survey conducted in a second interview that typically took place more than a year after the first interview (median time between interviews was 13.6 months). Non-responders include people who died during that period (3.1 percent of eligible adults), people who could not be located or contacted for the interview (3.0 percent), and people who refused to participate (3.4 percent). Only 0.2 percent are reported as not responding because they were incapable of self-response and no proxy was available (rules for the Phase II interview allowed proxies not

[4] This is the response rate to Phase II for people who responded to Phase I; household non-response to the NHIS core, which was 6.2 percent of households in 1995 (Botman, Moore, Moriarity, and Parsons, 2000) is not included.

residing with the individual, such as caregivers, to respond for an eligible adult). For a further 1.3 percent of eligible adults, no reason for non-response is recorded.

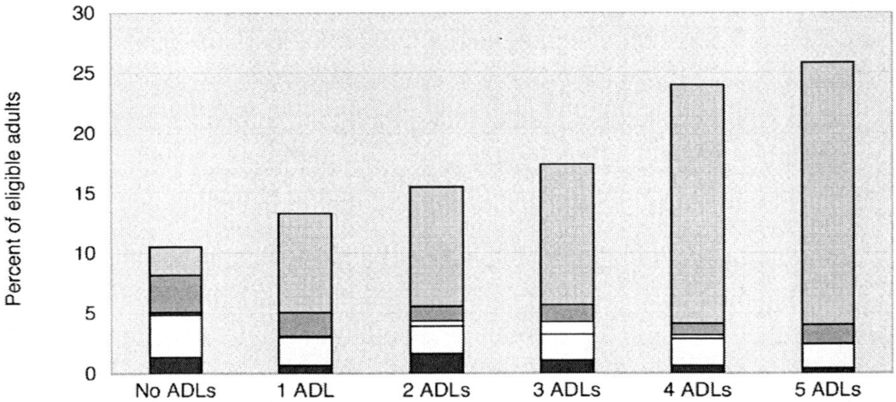

	No ADLs	1 ADL	2 ADLs	3 ADLs	4 ADLs	5 ADLs
Died	2.4	8.3	9.9	11.7	19.9	21.8
Can't contact	3.1	1.9	1.2	1.4	1.0	1.6
Unable & no proxy	0.2	0.1	0.4	1.1	0.3	0.0
Refused	3.5	2.3	2.3	2.1	2.2	2.0
Other/unknown	1.3	0.7	1.7	1.1	0.6	0.4

Figure 10.Reasons for non-response to NHIS-D PhaseII, by number of ADLs

The rate of non-response increases markedly with disability severity, as measured by the number of activities of daily living that a person gets help with (Figure 10). Only 10.5 percent of eligible adults with no ADL needs failed to respond to the survey, compared to 25.8 percent of people with all 5 ADL needs. However, closer inspection reveals that the increase in the non-response rate with the number of ADLs is due entirely to the greater mortality rate of people with greater ADL needs. Among people without ADL needs, 2.4 percent had died between Phases I and II, compared to nine times as high a fraction of people with 5 ADLs.

With the exception of mortality, which varies according to the impairment reported, non-response remains relatively low across impairment types.

The National Health Interview Survey 1997–2002, Sample Adult Section

For most of its history, the National Health Interview Survey was conducted entirely in the manner already described: Each household was contacted and all adults present at the time of the interview were invited to participate in answering questions about all members of the family. But in a major redesign of the National Health Interview Survey implemented in 1997, the family part of the questionnaire was shortened and much of the survey's content is now asked of only one randomly sampled adult per family. In families with children, information is also gathered about one randomly selected child through an interview with a knowledgeable adult. Although the change resulted in less information being collected from most households, the validity of that information was probably improved through the requirement that the sample adult respond to questions for himself or herself, with no proxies permitted.

The measures of activity limitation (for example, work, personal care, and home management), which are widely used to identify a population with disabilities in this survey, remain in the Family section, and continue to be answered by either self- or proxy response, depending on the availability, preferences, and ability of each adult respondent. However, new disability measures based on functional limitations were added to survey in 1997 and placed in the Sample Adult section. Only self-response was (and still is, in most cases) permitted to this section (National Center for Health Statistics, 2000); if self-response was not obtained for any reason, no sample adult information was gathered for the family. Unfortunately, the requirement of self-response resulted in levels of non-response to this section that are unusually high for the NHIS, and that varied from year to year as survey procedures were altered slightly. Self-response with assistance is not addressed in the NHIS field representatives' manual, nor is it recorded in the data set.

NON-RESPONSE TO THE SAMPLE ADULT SECTION

As shown in Figure 11, the non-response rate for all adults selected to respond to the sample adult section began at 10.2 percent when the survey was first fielded in the first quarter of 1997, and then grew more or less steadily to reach almost twice that level, 19.5 percent, by the end of 1999.[5] It would appear that, when the redesigned survey was initially fielded, the survey takers had not been fully trained in the necessity for self-response, and so proxy responses were still being accepted by some interviewers. Presumably, all the field representatives would have been fully trained, and the requirement of self-response reinforced by NCHS, by the third year of operation. Non-response drops substantially in 2000, when an exception to the no-proxy rule was introduced, and falls further in 2001, reaching a fairly steady level of about 16 percent.

These non-response rates above 15 percent compare very unfavorably to the 11 percent non-response rate for Phase II of the NHIS-D, which had the great disadvantage of a long period of time elapsing between interviews. In the case of the Sample Adult section, in contrast, the questionnaire is often completed in the initial family interview, and issues of people moving or dying are rare.

To better understand non-response to the Sample Adult section, it is useful to distinguish between two different scenarios: In one scenario, the family respondent—the person who took primary responsibility for identifying all the family members and answering the Family section of the survey—is randomly chosen to be the sample adult.[6] In the other, the sample adult is someone other than the family respondent.

[5] Again, this is non-response to the Sample Adult section among households responding to the Family section, and does not include household non-response of between 8.0 and 12.4 percent (National Center for Health Statistics, 2000, 2002).

[6] In families with only one adult, the sample adult is always the family respondent, and there is nothing random about it.

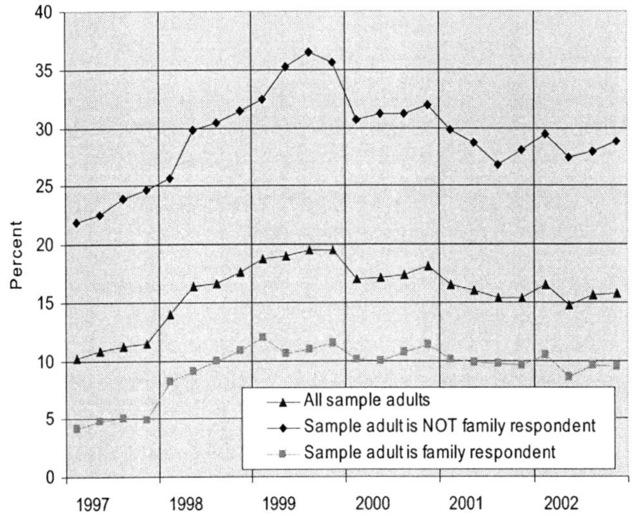

Figure 11. Non-response to the NHIS Sample Adult section among families responding to the core, 1997-2002

In the first scenario, in which the sample adult is the family respondent, the interview usually continues without interruption at the start of the Sample Adult section, and non-response hovers near 10 percent after rising from an initial rate of just under 5 percent (Figure 11). This case is not of particular interest for this analysis, because the family respondent has already established some level of capability and willingness to participate in the interview, and the level of non-response is not a true measure of the extent to which survey procedures accommodate and include people with disabilities.

When the sample adult is not the family respondent, however, the field representative must attempt to interview another person who may or may not be at home, be available to participate, or be able to participate in the survey in the form in which it is offered. Non-response rates are much higher when the sample adult and family respondent are different people than when they are the same person: initially at 21.9 percent and rising to above one-third of eligible respondents (reaching 36.5 percent in the third quarter of 1999), before falling back down below 30 percent in 2001. These very high levels of non-response reflect problems encountered when the survey taker must, in effect, begin a fresh interview with a new self-respondent.

SAMPLE ADULT NON-RESPONSE BY DISABILITY STATUS

As shown in Figure 12, people with disabilities, as defined by responses to the activity limitation questions in the Family section, have non-response rates that are roughly the same as, or a bit less than, people without disabilities during the first three years of the redesigned survey. In the figure, and throughout this section, the analysis is limited to the more relevant, second scenario in which the sample adult is not the family respondent.

Beginning in 2000, however, non-response rates for people with disabilities are lower than for non-disabled sample adults, especially in 2001 and 2002: 20.3 percent versus 29.3

percent in 2001 and 18.7 percent versus 29.6 percent in 2002. The reduction in non-response is due to a slight relaxation in the no-proxy rule introduced in 2000: “in a small number of cases, proxy responses are allowed if the selected adult had a physical or mental condition prohibiting him/her from responding” (National Center for Health Statistics, 2003). This “small number of cases” amounts to 2.9 percent of the sample in 2001 and 2002, with a dramatic effect on participation of people with severe disabilities, albeit by proxy.[7]

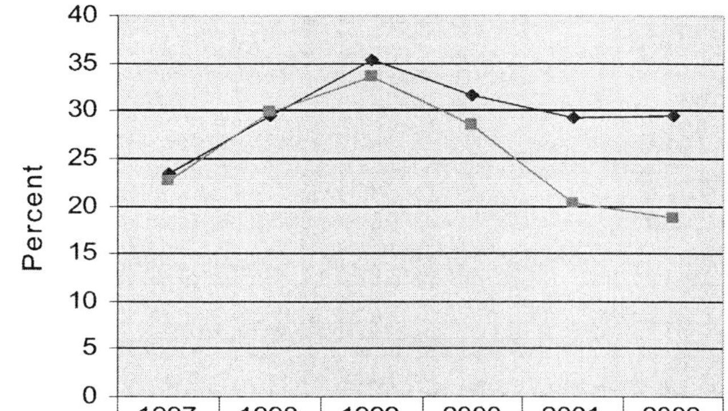

	1997	1998	1999	2000	2001	2002
No disability	23.3	29.5	35.3	31.6	29.3	29.6
With disability	22.6	29.9	33.5	28.6	20.3	18.7

Figure 12. Non-response to the NHIS Sample Adult section, for sample adults who are not the family respondents, 1997-2002.

To better compare non-response among those with and without disabilities, it is appropriate to control for demographic factors apart from disability status that might affect response rates. As we did for the NHIS-D, we construct logistic regression models controlling for age, sex, and educational attainment. Two models are constructed, one for the highest non-response years of 1999 and 2000 and the other for 2001–2002, during which proxy responses were permitted in certain cases.

Controlling for demographic factors, we find that non-response during 1999–2000 was significantly higher among people with disabilities, at 33.2 percent, than for those without disabilities, 30.5 percent. In 2001–02, non-response among people with disabilities drops dramatically to 20.1 percent, much lower than the corresponding rate for people without disabilities, 26.6 percent.

Again using the number of ADLs a person gets help with as a measure of disability severity, we find that non-response rates go up dramatically with severity in 1999–2000 (Figure 13). People with activity limitations but no ADL help needs have a non-response rate of 30.1 percent, not significantly different from the rate for those without disabilities, 30.4 percent. But with ADL needs come rising rates of non-response, ranging from 42.6 percent for 1 ADL to nearly two-thirds (64.1 percent) for 5 ADLs.

In 2001–02, however, there are no statistically significant increases in non-response with disability severity. People with 2 or 3 ADL actually have significantly lower non-response rates (of 9.7 and 11.5 percent, respectively) than people without disabilities (26.7 percent),

[7] Proxy response is not recorded in the NHIS public use file for 2000

controlling for demographic factors. The reintroduction of proxy response has made a world of difference in response levels, but self-response remains low: of sample adults in 2001–02 (who were not family respondents) who had 2 or more ADL needs, half (49.2 percent) responded by proxy (not shown in the figure and not controlling for demographic factors).

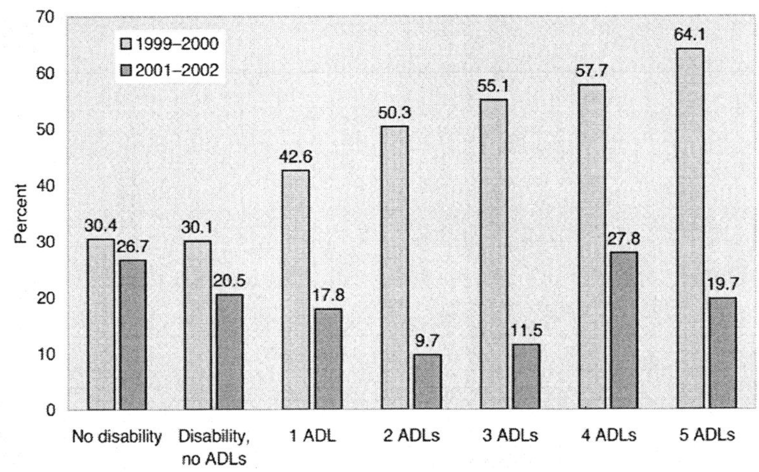

Figure 13. Non-response to the NHIS Sample Adult section, for sample adults who are not the family respondents, by number of ADLs and survey year, controlling for demographics

Because most of the functional measures of disability are contained in the Sample Adult section, we cannot use them to analyze response rates to that section. We instead make use of three items in the Family section: an ADL-like measure of need for help getting around the home (which was not counted as an ADL in the above analysis), a measure of difficulty walking, and a measure of activity limitation due to difficulty remembering or periods of confusion. Aside from that broad measure of cognitive impairment, we can construct a measure of severe cognitive limitation based on an indication of either senility/Alzheimer's or mental retardation as a cause of activity limitation. Other causes of limitation, from among the limited checklist now provided to respondents, do not yield significantly higher rates of non-response than for people with disabilities as a whole.

In models in which these four measures are included, along with the overall activity limitation measure, we find that people with severe mobility or severe cognitive limitations had high non-response rates in 1999–2000, at 48.0 and 44.4 percent, respectively, compared to 30.4 percent for people without disabilities and 28.6 percent for people with disabilities not related to mobility or cognition (Figure 14). People with non-severe mobility limitations are also significantly less likely to respond than people without disabilities, but there is no statistically significant difference for people with non-severe cognitive limitations.

In contrast, none of the differences that were significant in 1999–2000 remain significant in 2001–02, and people with non-severe cognitive limitations actually have a significantly lower likelihood of non-response than people without disabilities, 15.2 percent versus 26.7 percent. Again, this improvement in non-response rates is due mostly to proxy responses.

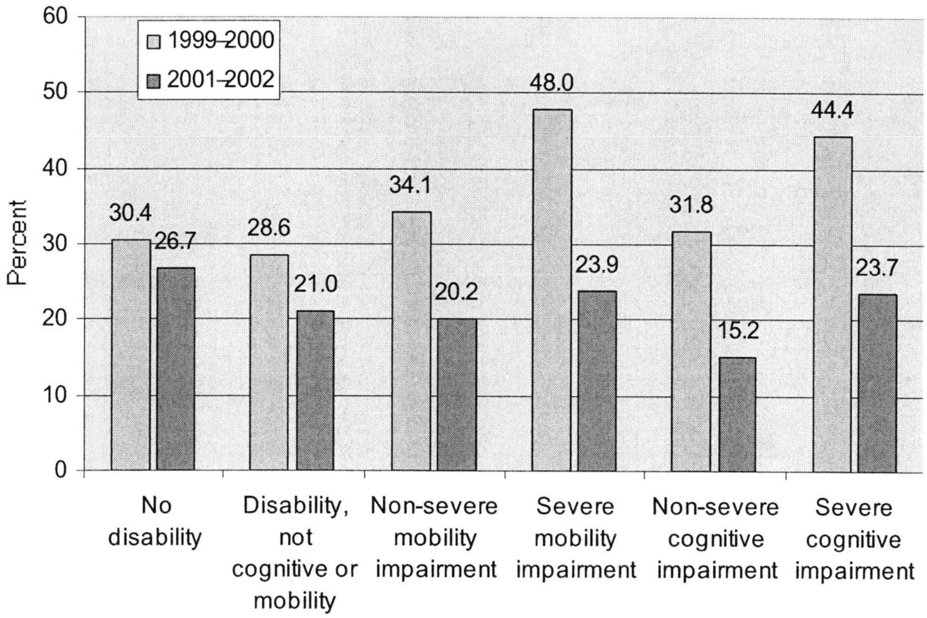

Figure 14. Non-response to the NHIS Sample Adult section, for sample adults who are not the family respondents, by impairment type, controlling for demographics

NON-RESPONSE BIAS IN THE FUNCTIONAL MEASURES

A good illustration of the consequences of high non-response rates, in particular among people with more severe disabilities, is found in the trend over time in the functional measures from the Sample Adult section (Figure 15). Although NCHS has provided sampling weights for the Sample Adult records that are designed to correct for non-response, there remain large year-to-year variations in rates of mobility, mental health, and sensory limitations that far exceed the standard errors of the estimates (indicated by error bars in the figure). Mobility limitation (any indication of difficulty in the nine measures of ambulation and upper body function) drops by 7 percentage points between 1997 and 1999, during which mental health limitation (any level of interference with daily activities by mental health symptoms) dropped by 5 points. Sensory limitations (any level of vision or hearing impairment) dropped by nearly 3 percentage points.

These huge changes cannot be real indicators of varying levels of impairment in the population. The activity limitation measures from the Family section (not shown) indicate no similar pattern of variation. Instead, the functional measures seem to roughly track the variations in non-response shown in Figure 11, with the lowest levels of all three functional measures occurring in 1999, the year of highest non-response, when few people with severe disabilities responded to the survey.

Unfortunately, the high and varying levels of non-response have rendered data from the NHIS Sample Adult section useless for disability-related trend analyses (Kaye, 2004), and data collected prior to 2001 are highly suspect for disability population estimates of any kind.

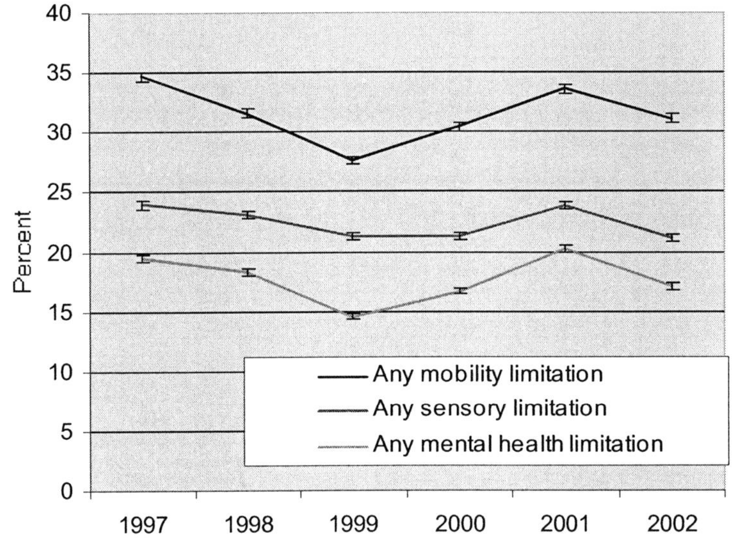

Figure 15. Proportion of adults limited in function, 1997-2002, based on responses to the NHIS Sample Adult measures.

DISCUSSION

It is clear that the best survey data are collected when a person responds for himself or herself, preferably in private and in an atmosphere conducive to truthful and accurate answers to questions that are sometimes personal or sensitive. At the opposite extreme is complete non-response, when no information whatsoever is collected for the person and for the thousands of similar people that the person was meant to represent.

In between are two types of response that are of intermediate value: assisted response, in which the person of interest responds with the help of someone else, typically a family member or caregiver; and proxy response, in which someone else (a family member or sometimes a caregiver) responds for the person without the person present. Of these, assisted response is clearly preferable, in that the person being sampled has an opportunity to answer at least some questions and correct any false statements made by their assistant. Proxy responses might be acceptable for certain types of information about which the proxy is knowledgeable, but its value is dubious when questions are of a subjective or more personal nature. Who would trust a proxy to answer this question from the NHIS Sample Adult section: "During the past 30 days, how often did [person] feel worthless?"

In this chapter, we evaluated the efficacy of two attempts to improve response validity by increasing self-response. One of these attempts was relatively successful: Phase II of the National Health Interview Survey on Disability achieved remarkably low non-response rates and, for its entire sample of people with disabilities, overall self-response rates that were substantially higher than the typical NHIS rates. However, people with more severe disabilities—in particular those needing help in activities of daily living or with severe cognitive, severe mobility, or any level of speech impairment—had unacceptably high levels of proxy response. Deaf people and people with mental health disabilities also had relatively high rates of proxy response.

In contrast to the relative success of the NHIS-D Phase II, the Sample Adult section of the annual NHIS failed, at least prior to 2001, in reliably collecting any information at all for people with the most severe disabilities. Though admirable in intent, the survey's absolute requirement of self-response, in the absence of a commensurate emphasis on accommodations, assisted response, and repeated attempts to interview people who were unavailable or temporarily unable, had an unfortunate and unintended consequence: high non-response rates overall, and especially high non-response rates for people with ADL needs or with severe cognitive or mobility impairments. Biases resulting from the exclusion of people with disabilities from the sample are evident in the year-to-year variability of the functional measures shown in Figure 15, making it impossible to detect trends in these measures over time.

Proxy response is better than nothing; when recorded as such in the data set, the researcher can decide for each item whether to trust a proxy or to ignore or impute the response. But it should be used as sparingly as possible. When proxy response to the Sample Adult section was permitted beginning in 2000, it was intended only for people deemed incapable of responding for themselves. This is clearly a subjective decision, and field representatives are no doubt tempted, upon hearing that an unavailable respondent has a disability, to declare the person incapable of response and then accept response from a proxy. Among people with severe disabilities whose response rates had been very low in previous years, proxy response became about as likely as self-response. Overall, non-response was lower for people with disabilities than for those without. The non-response problem had largely been solved, but at the expense of abandoning the worthy goal of greater self-response for this population.

Assisted response was not part of the interviewer training for the NHIS Sample Adult section, nor is there any indication in this data set when a person receives response assistance. In contrast, assisted response was permitted and recorded by the NHIS-D Phase II interviewers, but even there it was underutilized. For all types of impairments, levels of proxy response are far greater than those of assisted response. In clear cases in which a family member could have helped a person respond to the survey—for example, among people whose speech is difficult to understand outside the family but not within—the family member was far more likely to speak for the person than to facilitate self-response. A great many opportunities were missed to improve the quality of responses by including input from the person with a disability himself or herself.

Assisted response is consistent with the independent living model of disability, in which people are enabled, often through help received from others, to participate in home and community activities that would otherwise be closed off to them. Although it would generally be preferable to provide accommodations to enable all people with disabilities to self-respond without assistance, assisted response can be seen as a best practice for situations in which other accommodations are infeasible or insufficient, or when it is the person's preference. Even people with severe cognitive limitations are capable of answering some questions for themselves, especially subjective and evaluative measures, but better data may be collected when a family member assists with other items.

Self-response with assistance is clearly superior to response entirely by another person, and both are superior to no response. A way needs to be found in such surveys to foster pure self-response, encourage assisted response when truly necessary, and use proxies only as a last resort, after all other possibilities of accommodation, assistance, and perseverance have been exhausted.

ACKNOWLEDGMENT

This research was funded by the National Institute on Disability and Rehabilitation Research, U.S. Department of Education, under grant numbers H133B980045 and H133B03110.

REFERENCES

Andresen, E. M., Vahle, V. J., and Lollar, D. (2001). Proxy reliability: health-related quality of life (HRQoL) measures for people with disability. *Qual Life Res, 10*(7), 609-619.

Botman, S. L., Moore, T. F., Moriarity, C. L., and Parsons, V. L. (2000). *Design and Estimation for the National Health Interview Survey, 1995-2004.* (Vital and Health Statistics No. 2(130)). Hyattsville, MD: National Center for Health Statistics, Centers for Disease Control and Prevention.

Cynamon, M. (1994). National Health Interview Survey on Disability [Videocassette]. Hyattsville, Md.: National Center for Health Statistics, Center for Disease Control and Prevention.

Dorman, P. J., Waddell, F., Slattery, J., Dennis, M., and Sandercock, P. (1997). Are proxy assessments of health status after stroke with the EuroQol questionnaire feasible, accurate, and unbiased? *Stroke, 28*(10), 1883-1887.

Hendershot, G. E. (2003). *The Effects of Survey Nonresponse and Proxy Response on Measures of Employment for Persons with Disabilities.* Urbana-Champaign, Illinois: Disability Research Institute, University of Illinois.

Kaye, H. S. (2004). *Recent Trends in Disability Among Working-Age Adults* (Disability Statistics Center Working Paper No. 0401). San Francisco: University of California, San Francisco.

LaPlante, M. P., Kaye, H. S., Kang, T., and Harrington, C. (2004). Unmet need for personal assistance services: Estimating the shortfall in hours of help and adverse consequences. *Journal of Gerontology B: Social Sciences, 59*(2), S98-S108.

National Center for Health Statistics. (1998). National Health Interview Survey on Disability, Phase 1 and Phase 2, 1994 (machine readable data file and documentation, CD-ROM Series 10, No. 8A). Hyattsville, MD: National Center for Health Statistics.

National Center for Health Statistics. (2000). *1997 National Health Interview Survey Public Use Data Release: NHIS Survey Description.* Hyattsville, MD: Division of Health Interview Statistics, National Center for Heatlh Statistics, Centers for Disease Control and Prevention.

National Center for Health Statistics. (2002). *1999 National Health Interview Survey Public Use Data Release: NHIS Survey Description.* Hyattsville, MD: Division of Health

Interview Statistics, National Center for Heatlh Statistics, Centers for Disease Control and Prevention.

National Center for Health Statistics. (2003). *2001 National Health Interview Survey Public Use Data Release: NHIS Survey Description*. Hyattsville, MD: Division of Health Interview Statistics, National Center for Heatlh Statistics, Centers for Disease Control and Prevention.

Perry, J., and Felce, D. (2002). Subjective and objective quality of life assessment: responsiveness, response bias, and resident:proxy concordance. *Ment Retard, 40*(6), 445-456.

Rothman, M. L., Hedrick, S. C., Bulcroft, K. A., Hickam, D. H., and Rubenstein, L. Z. (1991). The validity of proxy-generated scores as measures of patient health status. *Med Care, 29*(2), 115-124.

Stancliffe, R. J. (1999). Proxy respondents and the reliability of the Quality of Life Questionnaire Empowerment factor. *J Intellect Disabil Res, 43 (Pt 3)*, 185-193.

Tamim, H., McCusker, J., and Dendukuri, N. (2002). Proxy reporting of quality of life using the EQ-5D. *Med Care, 40*(12), 1186-1195.

Todorov, A., and Kirchner, C. (2000). Bias in proxies' reports of disability: data from the National Health Interview Survey on disability. *American Journal of Public Health, 90*(8), 1248-1253.

U.S. Bureau of the Census. (1993). *Disability Followback Survey: Field Representative's Manual* (No. DFS-100 (1994)). Washington, D.C.: U.S. Bureau of the Census.

In: Towards Best Practices for Surveying People..., Volume 1 ISBN 1-60021-195-X
Editors: Thilo Kroll, David Keer et al., pp. 127-146

Chapter 8

NOTES FROM THE FIELD: CONTEMPORARY STRATEGIES FOR DEVELOPING SURVEYS OF PEOPLE WITH DISABILITIES: THE MASSHEALTH EMPLOYMENT AND DISABILITY SURVEY

Alexis D. Henry[1], Patricia Gallagher[2], Vickie Stringfellow[2], Leslie Olin[1], Fred Hooven[3], and Jay Himmelstein[1]

[1]Center for Health Policy and Research, Commonwealth Medicine, University of Massachusetts Medical School

[2]Center for Survey Research, University of Massachusetts Boston

[3]Center for Outcomes Research, University of Massachusetts Medical School

ABSTRACT

Health services and health policy researchers interested in the experiences and perceptions of people with disabilities commonly employ surveys as data collection tools. Yet, the best approaches to use in developing and administering surveys of people with disabilities have not been widely discussed in the literature (U.S. Department of Education, 2004). In this chapter, we describe the development and administration of the MassHealth Employment and Disability Survey (MHEDS), which was developed under the Massachusetts Medicaid Infrastructure Grant. The MHEDS was designed to gather information on disability and health status, employment status, and experiences with health care and other services among working age adults with disabilities enrolled in the state Medicaid program, called MassHealth. We discuss the key approaches that we used to define and refine the survey content and format, to conduct cognitive testing of the survey prior to fielding, and to administer the survey to nearly 3000 adults with disabilities in three MassHealth programs. In particular, we highlight the strategies that we used to involve multiple stakeholders, especially individuals with disabilities, in these development efforts. These approaches represent state-of-the-art strategies and can help ensure that the experiences and perspectives of people with disabilities are effectively captured.

THE MASSACHUSETTS MEDICAID INFRASTRUCTURE GRANT AND THE MASSHEALTH EMPLOYMENT AND DISABILITY SURVEY

The Massachusetts Medicaid Infrastructure Grant (MMIG) was funded by the Centers for Medicare and Medicaid Services and was jointly awarded to the Center for Health Policy and Research at the University of Massachusetts Medical School (UMMS) and the Massachusetts Executive Office of Health and Human Services' Office of MassHealth (Medicaid) in 2001. The primary goal of the MMIG has been to promote the competitive employment of working-age adults with disabilities in Massachusetts.

Funds for Medicaid Infrastructure Grants were mandated by the Ticket to Work and Work Incentives Improvement Act (The Ticket Act), signed into law by President Clinton in 1999. The Ticket Act was designed to encourage employment among people with disabilities by removing important work barriers. One oft-cited barrier is the concern that people with disabilities have that an increase in earnings will results in the loss of public health insurance provided by the Medicare and Medicaid programs (Hanson, Newman andVoris, 2003; Henry and Lucca, 2004; MacDonald-Wilson, Rogers, Ellison, andLyass, 2003). Two provisions of the Ticket Act addressed this issue. First, the Act extended the period of Medicare coverage for Social Security Disability Insurance (SSDI) recipients who continued to have a disability but no longer received cash benefits because of earnings from 4 years to 8 1/2 years. In addition, the Act encouraged states to develop or expand existing Medicaid Buy-in programs (Jensen and Silverstein, 2000).

Medicaid Buy-in programs allow individuals who qualify on the basis of disability but whose family income is too high to qualify for standard Medicaid (i.e. above 133% of federal poverty level [FPL]) to buy into Medicaid through premiums and other cost-sharing mechanisms. Prior to the Ticket Act, the Balanced Budget Act (BBA) of 1997 allowed states to develop Buy-in programs to provide coverage to working individuals with disabilities whose net family income was less than 250% of FPL. Under the Ticket Act, states could expand their buy-in programs to provide coverage to working individuals with disabilities whose income exceeds 250% of FPL. With the Ticket Act, states are free to set their own income limits, or to have no income limit at all (Ireys, White and Thornton, 2003).

States have used Medicaid Infrastructure Grants (MIG) funds to make changes in programs and systems to meet the needs of people with disabilities who want to work. Some states have used MIG funds to develop buy-in programs while others have improved access to their buy-in programs and to other services that support employment efforts among people with disabilities. Massachusetts is unique among states, because the Massachusetts buy-in program, known as the MassHealth CommonHealth program, predates both the BBA and the Ticket Act. The CommonHealth program, first implemented in 1988 and expanded during the 1990's, covers working age adults with disabilities with family income above 133% of FPL. To be eligible for the CommonHealth program, individuals must meet federal or state disability eligibility criteria. Individuals who work 40 hours per month or more are enrolled in CommonHealth Working and pay an income-adjusted premium payment. Those who are not working or work less than 40 hours per month are enrolled in CommonHealth Non-Working, must meet a one-time deductible based on family income, and also pay an income-adjusted premium. There is no income limit or asset test for the CommonHealth program.

Although Massachusetts has had a program available to working adults with disabilities for many years, until now little was known about individuals in the CommonHealth program regarding their disability or health status or regarding their employment experiences. The same was true regarding the experiences of individuals with disabilities in the MassHealth Standard program. Medicaid administrative data, primarily claims data, provide very limited information that can be used by researchers and policy makers to evaluate or to encourage enrollment into buy-in programs. One component of the Massachusetts Medicaid Infrastructure Grant (MMIG) has focused on trying to fill this knowledge gap. The monitoring and evaluation component of the MMIG[1] has been devoted to better understand the experiences of working age adults with disabilities enrolled in both the MassHealth CommonHealth and the MassHealth Standard programs. One of the first goals of the monitoring and evaluation component was to gather data that more fully described the experiences of working age adults with disabilities in MassHealth. The MassHealth Employment and Disability Survey was part of that effort.

Participatory Action Research

From the beginning, the activities of the MMIG have been informed by the perspectives of multiple stakeholders, including researchers, policy makers, service providers, and individuals with disabilities enrolled in MassHealth programs. Our efforts to understand the experiences and perspectives of these multiple stakeholders reflect our use of *participatory action research* (Whyte, 1991) approaches to guide many of the MMIG activities. Participatory action research, or PAR, refer to an approach in which researchers and the stakeholders whose lives or work may be affected by the research engage collaboratively in all phases of the research process, from the definition of the research question or problem through the interpretation, dissemination and utilization of research findings (Turnbull, Friesen and Ramirez, 1998). The use of PAR does not dictate the use of any specific research methodologies – both quantitative and qualitative methods can be implemented within a PAR framework. A PAR approach empowers participants who have traditionally been the "subjects" of research to directly influence the research process. Participants are valued for their insider perspective and their expertise with the research problem that is being addressed (White, Nary and Froehlich, 2001; Yeich and Levine, 1992). An important goal of a PAR approach is to create opportunities for research stakeholders to act as change agents, converting research findings into new policy, service or research initiatives.

It is not surprising that the disability field has embraced PAR strategies. The emergence of the disability rights movement and social models of disability in the past several decades has shifted the conceptualization of disability from primarily being a characteristic of an individual due to a medical condition to being a social construction, with disability largely

[1] The Massachusetts Medicaid Infrastructure Grant had three main components. In addition to monitoring and evaluation, grant funds were used to implement the CommonHealth Employment Connection, an information and referral service that provided information on CommonHealth and other employment support services for people with disabilities. The third component, the New England Partnership, provided technical assistance and support to other New England states with Infrastructure Grants.

being created by barriers in the environment. Accordingly, researchers have increasingly sought to understand the experience of disability from the perspective of the person in the context of his or her environment, requiring the participation of people with disabilities in research as informants and consultants (Brown, 2001). At the federal level, the National Institute on Disability and Rehabilitation Research (NIDRR) has advocated the use of PAR approaches in disability research for many years. The NIDRR long-range plan states,

> "The role of the disabled consumer in research is ... proactive and participative. Research must involve not only consumers but other stakeholders in understanding and interpreting research, in disseminating and applying research findings, and in planning, conducting and evaluating research (U. S. Department of Education, 2000, p. 13)."

Numerous authors have described the relevance of PAR approaches to a wide range of disability and health services research issues (e.g. Brown and Gordon; 2004; Nelson, Ochocka, Griffin and Lord, 1998; Taylor, Braveman and Hammel, 2004; Turnbull, et al., 1998). PAR strategies have been implemented in multiple ways. For example, in an evaluation of a supported education program for young adults with psychiatric disabilities, Danley and Ellison (1999) employed people with psychiatric disabilities as research assistants. Kielhofner and colleagues (2004) sought input from program participants to evaluate the effectiveness of and improve an employment program for adults with AIDS. A consumer-driven program for individuals with chronic fatigue syndrome involved people with chronic fatigue syndrome in planning and implementing services, as well as evaluating outcomes of the service (Taylor, Bravemen and Hammel, 2004). Robinson andKrauss (2003) involved family advisors as on-going consultants in a study examining experiences of families of children with disabilities and special needs in accessing health care services. PAR strategies have also been used to develop a web-based system for documenting outcomes of the national Assistive Technology Alternative Financing Program (Hammel, Finlayson and Lastowski, 2003). In recent years, researchers have begun to employ PAR strategies in the development of a variety of disability-related surveys and questionnaires (e.g. LaPlante, Kaye, Mullan and Wong, 2004; Lerner, et al., 2001; Rumrill, Roessler and Koch, 1999).

The use of PAR is not an "all or nothing" phenomenon. In discussing the application of PAR to research with families, Turnbull and colleagues (1998) described a six-level continuum of participation in research. At lower levels of involvement, stakeholders (e.g. individuals with disabilities, family members, providers) may act as research participants, advisory board members, or occasional consultants. At higher levels, they may act as on-going advisors, co-researchers or research leaders. The use of PAR strategies does not always require that those who are the focus of the research participate at the highest levels of involvement. However, Turnbull and colleagues argue that key to the implementation of a PAR approach is that the expertise of these individuals carries "equal or at least meaningful weight" (pg.183), and that they participate proactively, rather than only reactively commenting on decisions that the researchers have already made (Turnbull, et al., 1998).

Involving Stakeholders in Developing the MHEDS Content

We have found a PAR approach to be well suited to many of the MMIG activities, and have employed several strategies to involve stakeholders in the development of the MHEDS. Key stakeholders in the MMIG included:

- Representatives from the state Medicaid office (MassHealth);
- Representatives from other state agencies serving people with disabilities (e.g. the state vocational rehabilitation agency; the departments of mental health and mental retardation; the commission for the blind);
- Representatives from community-based provider agencies (e.g. independent living centers; psychosocial rehabilitation programs);
- MassHealth enrollees with disabilities;
- Researchers at the Center for Health Policy and Research;
- MMIG research consultants;
- Staff at CommonHealth Employment Connection, an information and referral service funded by the MMIG;
- The New England Partnership, a group of policy makers and researchers in other New England states with MIG grants.

With the awarding of the MMIG in 2001, two advisory groups were formed. The Consumer and Advocates Advisory Panel (CAAP) was comprised of representatives from the consumer, provider and advocates communities and the Interagency Advisory Group (IAG) was comprised of representatives of the various state agencies serving people with disabilities. In mid-2001, MMIG project staff conducted initial interviews and focus groups with members of these two groups in an effort to identify major barriers to employment for people with disabilities and to elucidate the role of health insurance and health care services in employment. While these discussions helped to make clear the complex challenges that people with disabilities face related to employment, particularly in terms of health insurance and health care, they also highlighted the lack of clear information about working age adults with disabilities in MassHealth programs that could be used by service providers and policy makers who serve people with disabilities in the state.

A MMIG core research team, responsible for carrying out the monitoring and evaluation activities of the grant, was formed in late 2001. Comprised of disability, health services and policy researchers, the research team included individuals with disabilities, including one individual who was enrolled in the CommonHealth program, individuals with family members with disabilities, and those with experience providing physical and mental health and employment services to individuals with disabilities. While the research team was comprised primarily of researchers located at the Center for Health Policy and Research at UMMS, researchers at other institutions served as consultants to all monitoring and evaluation projects. One of the first projects undertaken by the research team was the development of a survey that would gather baseline descriptive data on the disability, health and employment status of working-age adults with disabilities enrolled in both the MassHealth CommonHealth and the Standard programs.

Development of the MHEDS began in 2002. As a first step, the research team reviewed the data from the interviews and focus groups conducted with CAAP and IAG members, and reviewed existing surveys targeted to adults with disabling conditions concerning health, disability, employment, use of services, and experiences with Medicaid and other insurance programs. These efforts allowed the research team to begin to define the essential domains to be covered by the survey, to begin to identify potential survey questions, and to gain insights into the possible ways to structure questions. Two members of the research team were responsible for developing draft versions of the survey. Stakeholders in our advisory groups (the CAAP and IAG) were invited to participate in a survey work group. Facilitated by the two research team members, the survey work group reviewed multiple draft versions of the survey, suggested revisions to specific questions, and provided feedback on the length, language, clarity, order and relevance of the survey questions. Telephone conference calls and e-mail communication were the primary ways we conducted work group meetings, which provided multiple avenues for participation. The efforts of the survey work group were reviewed regularly by the research team, which met on a weekly basis. Draft versions of the survey were also reviewed by the MMIG research consultants, by New England Partnership researchers, by staff at the Office of MassHealth, and by two staff members at CommonHealth Employment Connection who were both enrolled in the MassHealth CommonHealth program.

As draft versions of the survey were developed, several of our stakeholders who were enrolled in MassHealth programs volunteered to participate in informal "pre-tests" of the drafts. The final draft version of the MHEDS was completed in early 2003. The survey covered six domains including experiences with MassHealth and other health insurance programs, disabling conditions and health status, activity limitations, employment and work-related activities, use of services, and demographics. The final draft version of the survey included a total of 124 questions, with sets of questions for both working and non-working respondents, as well as sets of common questions. Once this final draft version was completed, members of the research team worked with researchers at the Center for Survey Research at the University of Massachusetts - Boston, who completed cognitive testing of the draft survey, assisted the research team with revising and finalizing the survey, and administered the survey to adults with disabilities in three MassHealth programs. Cognitive testing, a more formal method for testing the quality of a survey instrument before fielding it, provided another opportunity for individuals enrolled in MassHealth to give input into the survey development process.

The Challenges of Using a PAR Approach

As have other researchers (e.g. Robinson and Krauss, 2003; Turnbull, et al., 1998), we found that there are challenges associated with using a PAR approach. Certainly, the collaborative nature of a PAR approach requires a time commitment from all involved. At the beginning of the project, the MMIG research team tried to ensure that stakeholders had the opportunity to learn from each other's experiences and perspectives by convening several advisory group (CAAP and IAG) meetings. As the survey development process got underway, we needed to ensure that stakeholders had sufficient time and opportunity to give input into the survey content and to review and respond to drafts of the survey as they were developed. The time needed for these reviews had to be balanced with the need to set reasonable deadlines in an effort to keep the survey development process moving forward.

One concrete challenge to managing the input of our multiple stakeholders was that satisfying everyone's interests meant that initially we had a survey that was much too long. Stakeholders also differed in their opinions about the complexity, order and language of certain survey questions. We were able to effectively address these challenges and reconcile differences through frequent discussions with our stakeholders about the goals of the survey, about ways to best make the survey "user-friendly" for our intended respondents, and by asking all stakeholders to consider their priorities and to make compromises. Sometimes all that was needed was for the stakeholders to learn the results of the empirical testing that contributed to instrument development – the cognitive interviewing and behavior coding described later in this chapter. Other times, stakeholders reached a compromise by talking through each of their apprehensions and finding common ground. Our efforts at good communication among all stakeholders allowed us to reduce the candidate items to a reasonable number by specifically addressing all of their concerns.

DEVELOPING CONTENT SUMMARY

We used multiple strategies, including individual interviews, focus groups, project advisory groups, structured work groups, and informal pre-testing of the survey to provide all stakeholders with opportunities to participate in the development of the MHEDS. The use of PAR strategies to develop survey content requires an investment of time, and cooperation and compromise, on the part of all involved. In the end, we believe these investments enhanced the quality of the MHEDS and the relevance of the data it has begun to yield.

Cognitive Testing: Respondents Helping to Refine a Survey

Cognitive testing is a powerful survey development tool. In cognitive testing, a nearly final version of the survey instrument is administered to members of the target population. These intensive individual interviews are used to monitor the cognitive processes of respondents as they answer candidate survey questions. Cognitive interviewing allows researchers to better understand individuals' in the target population comprehension of questions and how they go about answering questions. The goals are to identify proposed survey questions that are not consistently understood by the population of interest and to identify ways in which these items can be revised.

While an early method of inquiry into respondents' cognitive processes was proposed in the 1960's by Belson (1981), it was not until the first Cognitive Aspects of Survey Methodology (CASM) conference in the 1980's that cognitive interviewing became a key step in survey development (Presser, et al., 2004). Today, most major academic and governmental survey research centers, including the Census Bureau, the National Institutes of Health, and the National Center for Health Statistics, have cognitive interview “laboratories” to integrate respondent expertise and perspective into survey instruments. Cognitive interviewing allows researchers to learn if survey items are working as intended and to answer critical instrument development questions including: Will the proposed questions elicit valid information? Will respondents be willing to expend the effort required to provide useful information? Do the proposed survey items represent too great a respondent burden?

There are many ways that the survey response process can go awry. Respondents may misinterpret the questions, forget crucial information, make incorrect inferences from the information they retrieve from memory, or select an inappropriate response category. Cognitive testing allows the identification of problems that respondents may encounter during any of the four widely recognized components of the response process (Tourangeau, Rips and Rasinski, 2000):

- *Comprehension.* Do respondents attend to questions and instructions? Does the item represent a logical form of question? Can respondents identify what information the question is seeking?
- *Retrieval.* Can respondents retrieve the information necessary to answer the question accurately?
- *Judgment.* How well do respondents integrate the various pieces of information retrieved?
- *Response.* Are respondents able to appropriately map their judgment onto an appropriate response category?

Cognitive Testing Methodology

There are three principle approaches to cognitive interviewing. The first is *prospective* and involves "getting the story" from the respondent prior to administering the candidate survey questions. This approach allows interviewers to identify discrepancies and ask respondents to resolve any differences between the narrative they provided before the formal interview began and the responses they provide to the survey questions. Second is *concurrent "think-alouds"* where cognitive interview subjects are asked to verbalize their thought processes, as much as possible, as they formulate their responses to draft items. The third approach is *retrospective probing*, where subjects answer targeted questions about their thought processes, either immediately after an item is administered or at the end of the interview. In practice, cognitive interviewers are apt to use a combination of these three approaches. During cognitive interviews, interviewers often ask respondents to restate in their own words what they think a question is asking and to ask them why they chose a particular answer instead of other offered response options (Fowler, 2002). Frequently used probes include: What were you thinking while you answered that question? How did you come up with that answer? What does [term] mean to you? Did you know the answer, or did you have to guess? When did that [event] happen (Willis, 2004; Beatty, 2004)?

Cognitive testing can be used to evaluate both self-administered and interviewer-administered instruments. When testing self-administered questionnaires, such as mail or web-based surveys, cognitive interview subjects are asked to read some or all of the questions aloud. This allows researchers to evaluate the subject's ability to function effectively at the literacy level required by the draft instrument. With interviewer administration, the questions are read to the respondent to simulate a telephone or an in-person interview.

While cognitive testing is an extremely useful tool to test and develop survey questions, it is worth noting some limitations associated with the technique. Because cognitive testing is so time and labor intensive, the number of subjects involved is necessarily relatively small. Because the subjects may not be representative of the entire survey population, questions about the generalizability of the results can arise. In addition, because subjects are usually paid a monetary incentive for their participation, they may be more willing than unpaid respondents in real survey conditions to perform the cognitive work required to provide accurate responses. A final consideration is that different cognitive researchers may identify different problems and make different recommendations about the same set of questions (Groves, et al., 2004; DeMaio and Landreth, 2004).

Cognitive Testing of the MHEDS

There were many instrument development issues to take into consideration for the MHEDS. The target population was adults with a wide variety of mental and physical disabilities, and the sample would include both working and non-working individuals. A further complication was that the sample would include three sub-samples: individuals in the Standard MassHealth program, as well as those in two categories within the CommonHealth program, CommonHealth Working and CommonHealth Non-Working. While the coverage is similar, there are some characteristics (e.g. premiums, deductibles) that vary across programs. The research design for the survey called for dual mode administration; those who did not respond by mail would be contacted by telephone to be offered the opportunity to complete a telephone interview. Thus, the survey questions needed to function equivalently in both the mail and telephone interview versions. This was also a dual-language survey, with both Spanish and English versions of the instrument. Budget constraints were predictably also a consideration. The goals for the cognitive testing for MHEDS were to evaluate candidate survey items to see if they worked as intended, to identify logical and structural problems, problems for interviewers, and formatting issues.

Methodology

Senior staff members and specially trained cognitive interviewers at the Center for Survey Research (CSR) conducted one-on-one interviews in-person or by telephone. The interviews took 1.5 to 2 hours to complete and all participants were paid a $40 incentive. Interviewers followed a semi-structured protocol. The interview schedule included a set of test questions from the final draft version of the survey and a set of structured probes designed to understand how participants understood questions and went about answering them. The protocol called for interviewers to ask the test questions as worded, obtain answers to one or a short series of questions, and then proceed to the cognitive probes. Separate instruments were used for participants who were employed and for those unemployed. With participants' permission, interviews were audiotape recorded. Interviewers then used the tape recordings to later review the interview and record their observations. Both because there is great variation in people's abilities to successfully comply with a "think aloud" protocol and because some individuals in the target population were cognitively impaired, a decision was made to focus on a combination of the prospective and retrospective probing techniques.

Cognitive testing participants were selected to represent as diverse a group as possible with respect to gender, age, race/ethnicity, education level, and type of disability. The seven participants included Caucasian and non-Caucasian women and men, between the ages of 25 and 64, with both physical and mental disabilities. Participants' level of education ranged from 3rd grade to college graduate; three participants were currently employed.

Example of Item Development

To provide a concrete example of how cognitive interviewing informed item development, we focus now on a small set of items, submitted by the MMIG research team as candidate items in the final draft version of the MHEDS, that were intended to identify the respondent's primary disabling condition and the onset of disability. These items were adapted from items used in several existing surveys reviewed by the research team and stakeholders. We then go on to illustrate the changes made for cognitive testing, the report of the cognitive testing for these items, and finally the version of the questions revised on the basis of the cognitive testing that were ultimately fielded in the survey.

Proposed Disabling Condition and Onset Items

1) Please tell us which you consider to be your primary disabling condition. *(Mark only one.)*

   a) Musculoskeletal or orthopedic condition (such as back injury or pain, arthritis, or amputation)
   b) Neurological condition (such as spinal cord injury, multiple sclerosis, cerebral palsy, seizures, Parkinson's disease, or head injury)
   c) Mental health condition (such as depression, manic-depression, schizophrenia or anxiety)
   d) Cardiovascular or respiratory condition (such as heart disease, circulation problem, emphysema, cystic fibrosis or asthma)
   e) Sensory condition (such as deaf or hard-of-hearing, blindness or vision impairment)
   f) Mental retardation or other developmental disorder (such as autism)
   g) Alcohol or drug abuse
   h) Other: please tell us

2) Please tell us if your primary disability occurred *(mark only one):*
   a) At birth
   b) Suddenly and/or traumatically
   c) Progressively over time

As survey methodologists, we at the Center for Survey Research were concerned about the feasibility of administering the items as originally worded by either mail or telephone in the planned dual mode survey. We worried that many in the target population would find the level of literacy required by the multi syllabic and highly technical terms challenging. We also worried about the real risk that long response choices would overwhelm most respondent's short-term memory when the items were administered by telephone.

Given the wide range of disabling conditions in the MassHealth population, we thought that an open-ended version of the question would reduce respondent burden by allowing respondents to self-define their primary disabling condition. Their responses would be coded during data entry. The onset of disability item was broken into three separate questions such that respondents would be presented with a series of simple questions and skipped out of the series once the duration of their disability had been identified. These questions were planned to come late in the survey, beginning at question 90. The revised version of the items from the cognitive testing protocol follows:

Questions as Cognitively Tested

90. The next set of questions is about your disability and overall health.
    What do you consider to be your main disabling condition? [Open-ended]
91. Now we'd like to know when this disability was first diagnosed.
    Did this disability happen suddenly? Yes/No **[If YES, go to Question 94]**

If NO:

92. Did this disability happen slowly, over time? Yes/No **[If YES, go to Question 94]**

If NO:

93. Were you born with this disability? Yes/No **[If YES, go to Question 94]**

RESULTS OF COGNITIVE TESTING

There was a wide range of answers to the open-ended question regarding "main disabling condition". Of the five cognitive testing participants with mental problems, only two listed that as their main disabling condition (one of these also listed a physical condition – carpal tunnel syndrome). The other three listed physical problems – arthritis, replaced knee, trouble walking. When we cognitively probed this question and asked about how their health was when they first enrolled in MassHealth, we heard more about the mental illnesses. There are several possible reasons for this. First, for most people, the phrase "disabling condition" meant a physical condition. Also, mental illness is stigmatized and it is may be more socially acceptable to say one is disabled because of a physical problem. When a person has been on Medicaid for a long time, or has multiple physical and mental health problems, it could also be difficult to remember exactly what it was that qualified them for Medicaid (they also may not know what it was that qualified them, and this was not explicitly asked in the question). It became clear in the cognitive testing that the goal of the open-ended question on disability condition was not clearly defined. Were we asking about a current health problem, the original "qualifying condition" for MassHealth, or something else? A respondent who had a stroke and is now paralyzed on one side of his body said his "main disabling condition" is diabetes and high blood pressure (which he said caused his stroke). Did he answer correctly or should he have answered "stroke" or "I have trouble walking"?

The following recommendations were presented to the MMIG research team by CSR staff following the cognitive testing:

> Recommendation: Our recommendations will depend on the research goals for this item. If the goal is to learn what originally qualified respondents for MassHealth, we could try to ground the question more to when they first started receiving benefits. We also suggest that this question be asked earlier in the interview. In many cases the participants had already mentioned their disabling condition prior to having this item presented. When this question was asked, it threatened the rapport that had been built between the interviewer and participant; it made it appear that the interviewer was not attending to what the person was saying. We recommend moving these items toward the beginning of the interview, perhaps adding a phrase to link the health condition to the time when they qualified for MassHealth.

Based on the cognitive interview findings, the research team decided to move these items to the beginning of the instrument. The report also catalyzed a discussion between the MMIG research team and CSR staff about the research goals for identifying disabling conditions. Information on disabling conditions is not available in MassHealth administrative records. Initially we wanted to know about the "primary disabling condition." During the discussion about defining the goals for these items, we realized that some on the research team were interested in the condition that qualified the individual for MassHealth, others that wanted to know the most profound disabling condition, and still others that were interested in the first disabling condition in a respondent's life. The decision was made to use a series of easy to answer questions that would allow the respondent to identify multiple disabling conditions. The text of the items as fielded is presented below:

FINALIZED VERSION OF THE QUESTIONS AS FIELDED IN THE SURVEY

[1] People often get MassHealth or Medicaid for a disability or long-term health conditions, like problems with their physical or mental health. The next questions are about any disability or health condition you may have.

[2] Are you legally blind or deaf? [Yes/ No **If No, Go to #5]**

[3] 3. Were you born with this condition? [Yes/No **If No, Go to #5]**

[4] 4. Is this condition the result of an accident or injury? [Yes/No]

[5] 5. Do you have any physical disabilities that make it difficult for you to walk, move, or get around? [Yes/No **If No, Go to #8]**

[6] 6. Were you born with this disability? [Yes/No **If No, Go to #8]**

[7] 7. Is this disability the result of an accident or injury? [Yes/No]

[8] Do you have any mental or emotional problems, such as depression, anxiety, or bipolar disorder? [Yes/No]

[9] Do you have any type of developmental disability, such as autism or mental retardation? [Yes/No]

[10] Do you have problems with alcohol or drug use? [Yes/No]

[11] Do you have a disease or long-term illness such as cancer, heart disease, AIDS, or lung disease? [Yes/No]

[12] Do you have any disabilities or health conditions as a result of a serious head injury? [Yes/No]

The recommendations from the cognitive testing resulted in revisions to several other items. After revisions, the final fielded version of the MHEDS consisted of a total of 136 questions, with 122 questions for currently working respondents and 80 questions for currently non-working respondents.

COGNITIVE INTERVIEWING SUMMARY

Including individuals with disabilities in instrument development as cognitive interview participants played a significant role in improving the MHEDS. The survey instrument that emerged after testing was far more likely to collect meaningful data than any the research team could have created without the input of members of the target population. Candidate question wording does not always mean the same thing to respondents and researchers. It is well worth the effort to learn how potential respondents cognitively approach draft survey items. Even legacy questions from previous surveys may not be directly portable into new instruments. These items from previous surveys may not have been cognitively tested if they were developed and used prior to 1990. Even if the items were tested, the testing may not have been done with the population of interest in the new survey. Cognitive interviews are a cost effective and powerful tool for instrument development.

FIELDING THE MHEDS

Researchers at CSR administered a dual-mode survey (via mail and telephone) of adults with disabilities using final version of the MHEDS developed earlier in the project. The finalized instrument was translated into Spanish by a reputable academic translation service.

Sample

A sample of nearly 3000 individuals was randomly selected from all MassHealth members with disabilities, ages 19 to 64 who were enrolled for at least six months in either the CommonHealth Working (n=1000), CommonHealth Non-Working (n=952), or MassHealth Standard (n=1000) programs. Information from administrative records about sampled individuals included names, addresses, telephone numbers, dates of birth, and program enrollment.

Protocol for Dual-Mode Surveys

We followed a standard approach for administration of a dual-mode survey (Groves, et al., 2004). All sample members were sent an advance letter to provide information about the study goals and to inform potential respondents that participation in the survey was voluntary. The letter also included a telephone number to call if there were any questions. A standard mail protocol was then executed, which included mailing a questionnaire packet, a thank you/reminder postcard about a week later, and a replacement mailing to nonrespondents about 4 weeks after the initial mailing of the questionnaire packet.

Approximately two weeks after the second questionnaire packet was mailed, specially trained professional interviewers attempted to conduct telephone interviews with all sample members who had not responded by mail. The average length of the completed telephone interviews was just under 15 minutes. At minimum, 10 call attempts were made on weekdays and weekends, at different times of the day, in different weeks. The questionnaire was administered in a computer-assisted telephone interviewing (CATI) format.

In some cases, interviewers did not need to speak with sample members in order to enlist cooperation. Sometimes the messages left by interviewers on answering machines or with other household members served as reminders to sample members who then completed the self-administered questionnaire and returned it by mail. Everyone who mailed in a questionnaire was immediately removed from the list of nonrespondents so they would not be contacted again by telephone. All data were collected for this study between the last week of July and the fourth week of October 2003.

Challenges to Fielding the MHEDS

Steps to Ease Respondent Burden

In the advance notification letter and both questionnaire cover letters, we provided sample members with a number to call if they had questions or preferred to complete the questions via telephone interview. No additional mailings were sent to anyone who requested the telephone option. We also opted to accept any refusal, from either the respondent or a proxy, as a final refusal instead of attempting to convert those who refused into respondents. This step reduced the number of potential phone calls to the household, and in some cases, members who refused to speak with an interviewer later completed the self-administered questionnaire and mailed it back.

In order to accommodate potential respondents who tired quickly or had difficulty speaking or concentrating for prolonged time periods, the CATI program was set up to allow respondents to stop the interview at any point and return to the next question at a later date. This option for completing the questionnaire over the course of several short sessions proved helpful for people with physical or mental conditions that fount it difficult to complete the 15-minute interview in one sitting.

Strategies for Interviewer Briefing

Before telephone data collection could begin, all interviewing staff was briefed on the differences between the sample for this project and general population samples. We informed interviewers that some portion of the sample might include adults with developmental delay, cognitive impairments, or some form of mental illness. Emphasis was placed on the need for retaining the standardization of the interview process, e.g., being sure to read each question exactly as it was written. As with all other standardized interviews, there could be no extra clarification of terms, probing, or leading respondents to answer. On the other hand, interviewers were also reminded to be patient and not to rush respondents who needed time to think before responding.

One of the more delicate skills required of interviewers was the ability to redirect any respondents who tended to add tangential information or to ask non-survey related questions. We suggested that interviewers remind respondents that they would have the opportunity to add comments at the end of the interview, but needed to get through all the survey questions first.

Confidentiality Issues

There were two important pieces of information about each sample member that had to remain completely confidential throughout the data collection protocol. The first was that everyone in the sample received Medicaid benefits; the second was that each person has some kind of disability. In order to maintain the confidentiality of this information during the mailing phase, the envelopes in which the questionnaires were packaged did not include any information about the content of the instrument. The return address printed on the envelopes was that of the survey vendor rather than the Medicaid agency. Additionally, all correspondence was addressed to the sample member by name. During the telephone data collection phase, text was scripted for locating the sample member and leaving messages without any mention of either Medicaid or disabilities. This information was conveyed directly to the respondent once he or she was located.

Outcomes of Fielding the MHEDS

Phone Calls from Respondents

Following the mailings of the advance letter and questionnaire packets, we received a total of 61 phone calls from respondents or their proxies. The frequency and reasons for each call are presented in Table 1. Fifteen of the callers requested that an interviewer contact them by phone in order to complete the interview. For the other 46 cases, the data collection process was halted due to the information conveyed by the callers.

Table 1. Reasons and Frequency of Calls Made After Mailings

Outcome of Call	Frequency
Language problem	1
Extreme illness	3
Deceased	4
Cognitive disabilities	11
Refusal	27
Request phone interview	15
Total	61

Results and Response Rates

Table 2 shows the results of the mail and telephone data collection efforts. It can be seen that much better response rates were achieved with the two CommonHealth groups (65% and 69%) than with the MassHealth Standard group (40%)[2]. All three groups were fairly consistent in terms of the proportion of members who refused to participate, and refusals accounted for approximately 12% of the overall nonresponse.

Table 2. Final Results and Response Rates by Population

	CommonHealth Working	CommonHealth Non-working	MassHealth Standard	Total
Ineligible	6	13	12	31
Eligible	994	939	988	2921
Completed by mail	526	468	277	1271
Completed by Phone	160	139	120	419
Refusals	124	109	103	336
Other non-interviews	128	223	488	895
Response Rate*	69%	65%	40%	58%

* (Completed by mail + Completed by phone) / Eligible

However, a better picture of the reasons for nonresponse can be gleaned from Table 3.

Reasons for Nonresponse

Table 3 presents the breakdown of the cases listed in the "Other Non-Interviews" column in Table 2. It can be seen here that the largest source of nonresponse for all three populations was the inability to obtain a working phone number, either because none was listed or because one was listed but unpublished. For the CommonHealth Working group, the cases in these two groups combined to account for 43% of the overall nonresponse while 42% ended

[2] Response rates were calculated using the American Association for Public Opinion Research's (AAPOR) conservative RR1 formula (AAPOR, 2004).

the field period with no final result after 10 or more calls. For the CommonHealth Non-Working and MassHealth Standard groups, the inability to locate a phone number was by far greatest source of nonresponse. This problem is most obvious when the two CommonHealth groups are compared with the MassHealth group. For the latter, 68% of the overall nonresponse is explained by the lack of good contact information. Fully 34% of the total MassHealth Standard sample members could not be contacted by telephone for this reason. Based on these results, it can be seen that response rates were directly influenced by the quality of contact information obtained for each sample group.

Table 3. Breakdown of "Other Non-Interview" Final Results by Population

	CommonHealth Working	CommonHealth Non-Working	MassHealth Standard	Total
No phone number	58	69	273	400
Unpublished phone number	21	38	58	117
Foreign language	4	18	11	33
Extreme illness	7	14	17	38
Cognitive disabilities	17	13	30	60
Prolonged absence	--	2	5	7
No result after 10+ calls	77	69	94	240

SURVEY ADMINISTRATION SUMMARY

The perceived challenges to conducting surveys of adults with disabilities are not insurmountable. Perhaps the most important step is the question development process, including thorough testing of concepts and questions with members of the population of interest. In addition to the length and reading level of the final survey instrument, there are several points in the survey process where steps may be taken to reduce respondent burden. For example, the telephone number we included in our cover letters allowed sample members who had difficulty with the paper questionnaire to request that an interviewer contact them instead. Similarly, interviewers were prepared to conduct the interview over the course of several short sessions instead of a single telephone call with respondents who tired quickly or had other conditions that made a longer interview difficult.

Finally, our results indicate that the biggest impediment to achieving higher response rates is the lack of accurate contact information. Rather than being a problem unique to studies of adults with disabilities, this finding is similar to previous studies of the general population of publicly insured adults (Gallagher, Fowler, and Stringfellow, 2005). The 12% refusal rate obtained in this study is similar to that achieved in a previous health care survey of commercially insured adults (Fowler et al., 2002). It is especially important to note that while only 3% of sample members were unable to participate due to extreme physical or cognitive impairments, 18% of the sample could not respond due to the fact that current telephone numbers could not be obtained.

Conclusion

The strategies that we used to develop the MHEDS represent some state-of-the art approaches to survey development. Approaches that provide multiple opportunities for stakeholder input are particularly important when the goal of a survey is to understand complex phenomena such as relationships among disability, health and employment for people enrolled in a pubic health insurance program. These approaches resulted in a higher than expected response rate and have provided us with a wealth of data that we are just beginning to analyze. As these data are analyzed, we will continue to involve our stakeholders in interpretation and dissemination of MHEDS findings. Their input will be crucial to ensuring that the lessons learned from the MHEDS and other MMIG activities regarding the disability and employment experiences of adults with disabilities enrolled in Medicaid are useful to all stakeholders -- people with disabilities, service providers and policy makers -- both within Massachusetts and nationally.

Acknowledgements

The authors thank for following individuals for their contribution to the development of the MHEDS. At the Center for Health Policy and Research, Steven Banks, Bernard Bonsra, Jennifer Bowie-Katz, Allard Dembe, Lobat Hashemi, Ann Lawthers, Linn Morrel, and Susan Murray; at the Center for Survey Research, Carol Cosenza; at Abt Associate, Ray Glazier; the MMIG research consultants David Stapleton, Gina Livermore, John Butterworth, Pamela Hanes and Tina Edlund; at the Office of MassHealth, Ellie Shea-Delaney and Annette Shea; members of the New England Partnership; and members of the MMIG Consumer and Advocates Advisory Panel and Interagency Advisory Group. Development of the MHEDS and this chapter were supported by the Massachusetts Medicaid Infrastructure Grant (Grant # DHHS/11-P-91918), and the Massachusetts Medicaid and Comprehensive Employment Opportunities Infrastructure Grant CFDA # 93.768 (HCFA/11-91234). Funding for both Body Text + 14 pt, (Latin) Bold, Centered grants was provided by the Centers for Medicare and Medicaid Services.

References

The American Association for Public Opinion Research (AAPOR). 2004. *Standard Definitions: Final Dispositions of Case Codes and Outcome Rates for Surveys.* 3rd edition. Lenexa, Kansas: Author.

Belson, W. (1981). The design and understanding of survey questions. Aldershot UK: Gower.

Beatty, P. (2004). The dynamics of cognitive interviewing. In S. Presser, J. Rothgeb, M. Couper, et al., (Eds.), *Methods for testing and evaluating survey questionnaires.* (pp. 45-66). Hoboken, NJ: John Wiley and Sons, Inc.

Brown, S. C. (2001). Methodological paradigms that shape disability research. In G. L. Albrecht, K. D. Seelman and M. Bury (Eds.), *Handbook of disability studies.* (pp. 145-170). Thousand Oaks, CA: Sage Publications.

Brown, M. and Gordon, W. A. (2004). Empowerment in measurement: "Muscle," "voice," and subjective quality of life as a gold standard. *Archives of physical medicine and rehabilitation*, 85 (4, Supplement 2), S13-S20.

Danley, K. and Ellison, M. L. (1999). *A handbook for participatory action researchers.* Boston, MA: Center for Psychiatric Rehabilitation, Sargent College of Health and Rehabilitation Sciences, Boston University.

DeMaio, T. J. and Landreth, A. (2004). Do different cognitive interview techniques produce different results? In S. Presser, J. Rothgeb, M. Couper, et al., (Eds.), *Methods for testing and evaluating survey questionnaires.* (pp. 89-108). Hoboken, NJ: John Wiley and Sons, Inc.

Fowler, F.J. (2002). *Survey research methods.* Thousand Oaks, CA: Sage Publications, Inc.

Fowler, F. J., Gallagher, P. M., Stringfellow, V. L., Zaslavsky, A. M., Thompson, J. W., and Cleary, P. D. (2002). Using telephone interviews to reduce nonresponse bias to mail surveys of health plan members. *Medical Care*, 40 (3), 190-200.

Gallagher, P. M., Fowler, F. J., and Stringfellow, V. L. (2005). The nature of nonresponse in a Medicaid survey: Causes and consequences. *Journal of Official Statistics*, 21(1), 73-87.

Groves, R. M., Fowler, F. J., Couper, M. P., Lepkowski, J. M., Singer, E., and Tourangeau, R. (2004). *Survey methodology.* Hoboken, NJ: John Wiley and Sons, Inc.

Hammel, J. Finlayson, M., and Lestowski, S. (2003). Using participatory action research to examine outcomes and effect systems change in assistive technology financing. *Journal of Disability Policy Studies*, 14, 98-108.

Hanson, K., Neuman, T., and Voris, M. (2003). *Understanding the health-care need and experiences of people with disabilities.* Melno Park, CA: The Henry J. Kaiser Family Foundation.

Henry, A. D., and Lucca, A. (2004). Facilitators and barriers to employment: The perspectives of people with psychiatric disabilities and employment service providers. WORK: *A Journal of Prevention, Assessment, and Rehabilitation*, 22, 169-182.

Jensen, A., and Silverstein, R. (2000). *Improvements to the SSDI and SSI work incentives and expanded availability of health care services to workers with disabilities under the Ticket to Work and Work Incentives Improvement Act of 1999.* Policy Brief, Volume 2, Number 1. Center on State Systems and Employment Outcomes, Institute for Community Inclusion/UAP, Center for Workforce Investment and Employment Policy, Community Options, Inc.

Kielhofner, G., Braveman, B., Finlayson, M., Paul-Ward, A., Goldbaum, L and Goldstein, K. (2004). Outcomes of a vocational program for people with AIDS. *American Journal of Occupational Therapy*, 58, 64-72.

LaPlante, M. P., Kaye, H. S., Mullan, J., and Wong, A. (2004). Including people with disabilities in questionnaire development: An example of a best practice for improving validity of survey measures. Paper presented at the Workshop on Best Practices for Surveying People with Disabilities. Washington DC: Interagency Committee on Disability Research.

Lerner, D., Amick, B. C., Rogers, W. H., Malspeis, S., Bungay, K., and Cynn. D. (2001). The work limitations questionnaire. Medical Care, 39, 72-85.

MacDonald-Wilson, K. L., Rogers, E. S., Ellison, M. L., and Lyass, A. (2003). A study of the social security work incentives and their relation to perceived barriers to work among persons with psychiatric disability. *Rehabilitation Psychology*, 48, 301-309.

Nelson, G., Ochocka, J., Griffin, K., and Lord, J. (1998). "Nothing about me without me": Participatory action research with self-help/mutual aid organizations for psychiatric consumer/survivors. *American Journal of Community Psychology,* 26, 881-912.

Presser, S., Couper, M. P., Lessler, J., Martin, E., Martin, J., Rothgeb J., and Singer, E. (2004). Methods for testing and evaluating survey questions. In S. Presser, J. Rothgeb, M. Couper, et al., (Eds.), *Methods for testing and evaluating survey questionnaires.* (pp. 1-22). Hoboken, NJ: John Wiley and Sons, Inc.

Robinson, D. and Wyngaarden Krauss, M. (2003). Lessons from the field: Participatory action research in a family research project. *Mental Retardation,* 41, 460-464.

Rumrill, P. D., Roessler, R. T., and Koch, L. C. (1999). Surveying the employment concerns of people with multiple sclerosis. A participatory action research approach. *Journal of Vocational Rehabilitation*, 12(2) 1999, 75-82.

Taylor, R. R., Braveman, R. and Hammel, J. (2004). Developing and evaluating community-based service through participatory action research: Two case examples. *American Journal of Occupational Therapy*, 58, 73-82.

Tourangeau, R, Rips, L. J., and Rasinski, D., (2000). *The psychology of survey response.* Cambridge, UK: Cambridge University Press.

Turnbull, A.P., Friesen, B.J., and Ramirez, C. (1998). Participatory action research as a model for conducting family research. *Journal of the Association for Persons with Severe Handicaps, 23* (3), 178-188.

U. S. Department of Education (2004). Workshop on best practices for surveying people with disabilities. Washington, DC: Interagency Committee on Disability Research.

White, G. W., Nary, D. E. and Froehlich, A. K. (2001). Consumers as collaborators in research and action. *Journal of Prevention and Intervention in the Community*, 21(2), 15-34.

Whyte, W. F. (1991). Participatory action research. Newbury Park, CA: Sage Publications, Inc.

Willis, G. (2004). *Cognitive interviewing: A tool for improving questionnaire design.* Sage Publications, Inc: Thousand Oaks, California

Yeich, S. and Levine, R. (1992). Participatory research's contribution to a conceptualization of empowerment. *Journal of Applied Social Psychology*, 22, 1894-1908.

In: Towards Best Practices for Surveying People…, Volume 1 ISBN 1-60021-195-X
Editors: Thilo Kroll, David Keer et al., pp. 147-164

Chapter 9

INITIAL DEVELOPMENT OF THE DISABILITY AND ACTIVITY IMPACT SCREENER (DAIS): AN EXAMPLE OF QUALITATIVE MEASUREMENT DISCOVERY

Mitchell P. LaPlante, H. Stephen Kaye, Joseph T. Mullan, and Alice Wong
Disability Statistics Center
Institute for Health and Aging
University of California, San Francisco

ABSTRACT

Survey measures of disability have been developed without sufficient consideration of how people with disabilities see themselves, and are focused negatively on what people cannot do or have difficulty with doing. The validity of that approach has been seriously challenged. We conducted a series of focus groups with over one hundred participants to explore how people with disabilities think about disability in their daily lives. Transcripts were analyzed independently by three researchers to identify common themes. People with disabilities are more concerned with how they do things differently, and the problems they encounter in doing so, rather than what they cannot do or have difficulty doing. Doing things differently included using personal assistants, assistive technology, taking more time, and avoiding or minimizing physical and social barriers. We developed a new instrument, the Disability and Activity Impact Screener (DAIS), to capture these ideas. It is possible to identify people with disabilities by focusing on differences in the ways that people perform day-to-day activities. This approach is positively oriented, is more consistent with how people with disabilities view themselves, and is potentially more valid. Including people with disabilities from the start of instrument development can lead to more valid questionnaire items and measures and is recommended as a best practice.

INTRODUCTION

While substantial progress was made in health and disability measurement during the twentieth century, no global measure has yet been developed that is universally regarded as a good way to identify populations with disabilities. The lack of valid, practical, and well understood survey measures for identifying people with disabilities and assessing their experiences has hindered data collection and delayed a full understanding of the factors that influence the participation of people with disabilities in society. To date, most survey questions on disability have been developed without the involvement of people with disabilities and have been firmly based on a medical model, in which disability is seen as arising solely from a health condition or impairment, without regard to the social and physical environments.

The specific goals of the research we report in this chapter involve a qualitative measurement discovery process using focus group discussions: 1) to identify important themes in the lives of people with either self-identified disabilities or some difficulty performing daily activities, and 2) to examine the language used by them to describe their lived experiences, of their bodies as well as their social and physical environments. By using themes and language expressed by people with disabilities themselves, our ultimate goal is to develop a set of survey questions that can more accurately identify the population with disabilities and more adequately address their diverse experiences and activities.

The two main approaches toward measuring disability currently in use are based on conceptual frameworks of outmoded utility given current conceptions of disability. The activity limitation approach, in which survey respondents are asked about difficulties or inabilities in performing certain age-typical activities, fails to recognize stigma, barriers in the physical environment, and institutional discrimination as sources of problems for people with disabilities (Scotch and Shriner, 1997). The functional limitation approach, in which respondents are asked about difficulties performing basic functions such as walking, seeing, or hearing, fails to recognize the degree of variation in function that exists amongst individuals and casts a large net around functional problems that often have little consequence for people in their day-to-day lives. Both approaches focus on limitations and difficulties rather than adaptations and accommodations that allow people with disabilities to act at a higher level.

The United States Commission on Chronic Illness (1957) used a measure of disability based on how a health condition or impairment limits a person's recreational and role activities. That measure has been employed in the National Health Interview Survey since 1969 to identify people with disabilities and has been adopted in many other surveys since. However, many people with disabilities view their activities as being limited by physical and social barriers in their environments, not by their health or impairments. Thus, people with disabilities do not always endorse questions about activity limitations, leading to false negatives.

In the functional limitation approach, questions focus not on complex activities but on basic human functions, in which the environment plays less of a role, rendering the omission of environmental influences less problematic. However, people are not all created equal, making it hard to determine at what point is a functional difficulty becomes a disability. When many people report some difficulty lifting a 25 pound bag of groceries, is that a sensible measure of disability? Without attention to reasonable selection of functional items and severity thresholds, the functional approach may include too many people as having disabilities, many of whom would not perceive themselves as having a disability, and can lead to false positives.

Recent theoretical models have argued that we need to locate the concept of disability in a broad view of human functioning, so that it is possible to identify the key aspects of the phenomenon and measure them adequately. These theoretical expansions have attempted to develop models that view disability as a complex outcome of personal, social, and environmental factors, and that avoid some of the obvious negative connotations of earlier models (Bickenbach, Chatterji, Bradley, and Ustun, 1999; Fougeyrollas and Beauregard, 2001; Gray and Hendershot, 2000). Unfortunately, these more complex models have not been operationalized (Altman, 2001) and, despite the theoretical advances that have occurred, national surveys continue to use measures based on the biomedical model (Fujiura and Rutkowski-Kmitta, 2001; Hahn and Hegamin, 2001).

Because so much measurement has been derived from the biomedical and functional limitation models, there is little systematic research that informs us of the way that the social and physical environments shape disability. Because measures have not kept pace with theory, it is impossible to evaluate empirically competing models. Most important, we suspect that existing measures are not meaningful to the people they purport to describe or their lived experiences of disability (Gill, 2001; Hahn and Hegamin, 2001). We suspect that they are often not adequate reflections, because they identify people in terms of activities or functions that people cannot perform, or have difficulty performing, perpetuating negative images of people. These measures ignore people's lived experiences, and the ways they participate in society within their social and physical contexts. In brief, the current survey measures focus on what people cannot do rather than on what they actually do or could do under certain conditions.

The need for better disability measures is critical: The U.S. Census Bureau, in the past 8 years, has counted from 39 to 54 million people as having a disability. (McNeil, 2001; Stern, 2003; Stern and Brault, 2005), casting doubt on the accuracy with which the nation allocates funds and opportunities to people with disabilities. The Bureau of Labor Statistics (BLS) has been tasked to design and implement a statistically reliable and accurate method to measure the employment rate of adults with disabilities, pursuant to Presidential Executive Order 13078. However, initial work by the BLS indicates that available survey measures have serious problems (US DOL, 2005).

As a result of such measurement issues, valuable information goes uncollected as survey developers refrain from including questions on disability in general-purpose surveys. For too long, Federal surveys have been fielded without disability measures—or with measures too readily subject to criticism—resulting in a lack of reliable statistics on the population with disabilities in key areas, such as housing, employment, political participation, and social participation. Furthermore, those surveys that do identify a population with disabilities do so in terms of activities or functions the person cannot perform or has difficulty performing, perpetuating negative images of people with disabilities as being unable to participate in society, rather than as people who do participate, though in a different way than most other people. Something better is needed, a way of measuring disability that is appropriate to the way in which people with disabilities go about living their lives.

In this chapter, we describe our efforts to develop a new approach to identify people with disabilities in surveys. A qualitative measurement discovery process was undertaken, one that engaged people with disabilities about how disability impacts their day to day lives. We chose to begin with focus group discussions because they are flexible and particularly useful to develop a map of participants' experiences; that is, to generate rather than to test hypotheses. When focus groups are working well, the participants are active collaborators in the research, describing their experiences in their own language, and stimulating others in the group to discuss topics they might not have considered. Focus group discussions may also provoke us, the researchers, to consider new ways of conceptualizing an area (Kitzinger, 1994; Morgan, 1997). The use of focus groups is consistent with a call for the inclusion of target populations in the development and assessment of measures in health outcomes research (Stewart and Napoles-Springer, 2000; McHorney, 2003). This call for inclusion of target populations is especially important in research on disability because people with disabilities are often not included in research and often not consulted about important dimensions of their experience (Hahn and Hegamin, 2001; Meyers and Andresen, 2000; O'Day and Killeen, 2002). Because it is the nation's goal that people with disabilities live more independently and participate more fully in society, the activity and functional limitation approaches need to give way to a new approach that recognizes how people with disabilities actually participate in the world.

Through this qualitative measurement discovery process, people with disabilities suggested new concepts leading to the construction of promising new items for measuring disability. We suggest qualitative measurement discovery as a best practice for discovering new ways to identify people with disabilities in surveys and recommend its use in improving the relevance of survey questions on disability more generally.

EXISTING DISABILITY MEASURES

National surveys that attempt to identify people with disabilities generally use one of two approaches, neither of which is well suited to the task of identifying a clearly delineated population, defined in a way that is relevant to current conceptions of disability. The activity limitation approach, exemplified by the National Health Interview Survey (NHIS), involves asking respondents whether a health condition or impairment prevents or limits their participation in their major activity—an age-appropriate activity such as play or school for children, work or housework for non-elderly adults, and personal care and home management for elderly persons—or whether they are limited in other activities. The functional limitation approach, most extensively used in the Survey of Income and Program Participation (SIPP), consists of a lengthy series of questions on functional difficulties in various dimensions, such as hearing, vision, mobility, cognition, and mental health. In both approaches, people reporting any limitation are generally regarded as having disabilities, with severe disability defined as an inability to perform either the major activity or one or more of the functions.

Other surveys use a subset of one or the other approach, or a combination of the two. The Current Population Survey has a question on work limitation, a key component of activity limitation. The 2000 decennial Census and the American Community Survey use an abbreviated set of essentially functional questions, along with two questions on activity limitation—one on personal care activities and another on work.

Both the activity and functional limitation approaches are firmly rooted in the medical model, in which disability is seen as arising solely from characteristics of the individual, such as a health problem, impairment, or functional difficulty, rather than from an interaction between the individual and the environment. Thus, the NHIS asks working-age adults whether "any impairment or health problem" keeps them from working, disregarding the possibility that they may be prevented from working largely because employers won't hire them or give them accommodations or because workplaces or transportation systems are inaccessible to them. The functional approach aims to avoid environmental concerns by focusing on problems in performing certain functional tasks, thus distancing itself even further from the activities a person may or may not engage in, from the barriers and facilitators that could inhibit or enable a person with a disability to live independently.

In the functional approach, any difficulty in any aspect of function is assumed to be in some way disabling. But the lack of any kind of measure of the impact of these difficulties on daily life results in an overly broad measure of disability, including many people who seem to be affected only minimally by their limitations, if at all. For example, of the 10.4 million working-age adults identified in the SIPP as having non-severe disability in 1997, 82.0 percent were employed, a rate only slightly below that of their non-disabled peers (84.4 percent; McNeil 2001).

Both approaches suffer weaknesses with regard to insufficient testing and validation of the questions. We do not know what people mean when they say they are limited "in any way in any activities": Are these important or trivial activities, and are the limitations substantial? Nor do we really understand why a consistent 15 percent of people prevented "from working at a job or business" report that they are employed at the time of the interview. As for the functional approach, even the 50 questions on function in the SIPP fail to capture all of the people we would regard as having disabilities: For example, people disabled by chronic pain, poor stamina or low energy, general ill health, or disfigurement, though perhaps very limited in activity or subject to high levels of discrimination, would not necessarily be covered under any of the functional categories. We also have no way of knowing whether an inability in one dimension—say deafness or blindness—is equivalent in impact to an inability in another area—say walking one-quarter mile.

Finally, the functional and activity limitation approaches share a common perspective in that they both focus on the tasks and activities that people with disabilities cannot do or have difficulty performing, rather than the tasks and activities that people can and do perform. Continuing to define a population according to their inabilities—whether to work or to walk, to attend a regular class or read a newspaper—perpetuates negative images of people with disabilities as people who are unable, rather than as people who are able to engage in many activities, and frequently do so, but often in different ways than other people.

The aim of correcting these weaknesses is the starting point of our work in developing new survey questions to define a population with disabilities. We believe that, by including the perspective of people with disabilities in all aspects of this effort, we gain a significant advantage over the previous approaches described above.

Data And Methods

Over a two year period, from 2000-2001, we conducted thirteen focus groups of people in the San Francisco metropolitan area with various types of disabilities, comprising 86 participants, who were encouraged to speak about the meaning of disability in their daily lives. Eight of the groups were heterogeneous, composed of individuals with a variety of sensory, physical, cognitive, or emotional difficulties, and five were homogeneous. These included a group of persons who were hard of hearing, a group of Deaf users of American Sign Language, a group with mobility impairments, a group with visual impairments, and a group with obsessive-compulsive disorders. Together, they represented the broad range of persons with disabilities, including both working age adults and seniors, equal numbers of men and women, and ethnic diversity, including African Americans, Asians, Pacific Islanders, and Latinos.

Recruitment approaches varied with the specific group, but typically involved making contact with local organizations, mailing letters, distributing flyers, and sending email descriptions of the study. Participants were paid $25 for the two hour sessions, and were reimbursed for transportation costs and an attendant, if needed. Consent forms in alternative format (e.g., Braille or on tape) were made available. We included real time captioning for the hard of hearing group and ASL interpreters for the Deaf group, and we conducted one group in Spanish.

Questions

After describing the research objectives, we told participants that we were interested in how they describe themselves, their experiences, and their surroundings. Because our focus was on how participants experienced their day-to-day lives, we never directly asked them to describe their biomedical conditions. We asked a series of open-ended questions (and follow-up questions) regarding participants' definitions of disability and their experiences of their social and physical environments. Although the exact questions we asked varied by group, we covered the following three broad areas in each group.

The meaning of disability:

1. What makes you think that you are disabled, or not disabled?
2. What do you think of when you hear the word 'disabled?'

Physical Barriers

1. What conditions in your physical world make it difficult to do what you want to do?
2. How would you describe the problems that you have with your physical surroundings as you go about doing things in your everyday life?

Challenging Situations

1. What situations make you aware of your difficulties or disability?
2. When do you NOT feel disabled?

We encouraged the participants to help guide the direction of the discussion, to feel free to talk with each other, and to bring up important ideas not raised by the facilitator. Participants were quite interested in answering the questions, and, without much prompting, talked freely. Generally, we were able to ask only about two or three general questions (with follow-up prompts) during a two-hour session. We tried to remain flexible and to follow the flow of discussion within each group. For example, a follow-up prompt to a general question about physical barriers might involve asking for instances of challenging situations people encountered.

A transcribed audiotape of each discussion was analyzed by two coders (JTM and AW), who developed and refined their categories throughout the data collection process. Each focus group discussion was broken down into segments of a participant's speech, which is a relatively uninterrupted set of sentences. Each speech was subdivided into meaningful codeable segments. Coding of these smaller segments was conducted independently by the two coders. The research team then collaboratively worked to synthesize the smaller codes into larger segments that formed coherent and meaningful patterns. The themes outlined below emerged through an iterative process of analysis and synthesis, as the team moved back and forth between the speeches, codes, and larger thematic patterns (Glaser and Strauss, 1967).

THEMES FROM THE DISCUSSIONS

Six themes stand out as salient dimensions of the discussions. Three of these we refer to as Major Themes, because they appeared consistently across groups, provoked energetic discussion, provided links to other themes, and helped form a conceptual map of participants' experiences.

Striking similarities were found across groups in the topics that were discussed, in particular in three key areas:

- Doing things differently, including use of special equipment or personal assistance, engaging in activities at a slower pace or taking longer to do things, and finding alternative strategies to perform activities that other people may do without difficulty.
- Problematic social interactions, such as people staring at, avoiding or excluding individuals, or treating them in a patronizing or otherwise inappropriate way. Barriers in the social environment were a much more frequent and heated topic of conversation than barriers in the physical environment. These barriers often occur as the result of doing things differently, but can also be the reason a person chooses to do things differently.
- Management strategies, including careful planning of activities to avoid potential barriers or poor treatment, planning for contingencies in case barriers or problems are encountered, and selection and prioritization of activities so that the most important get done in the limited time or with limited stamina.

Three additional common themes were also noted:

- Problems in the physical environment, generally involving mobility or communication barriers. Although a less frequent topic of discussion than anticipated, physical barriers did present problems, often in combination with social barriers.
- Difficulties in personal functioning, including chronic pain, ill physical or mental health, and lack of stamina. Despite the importance of the physical and social environment in causing disability, many people with disabilities attribute their lack of participation to causes related to bodily or mental function rather than to the environment.
- The "work of disability," or the time and energy expenditures associated with the first three themes, such as that of smoothing out difficult social interactions, of having to do extra planning in case of physical barriers, of finding alternative ways of getting things done. This indicates an awareness that people with disabilities must deal with tasks and situations that are not experienced by people without disabilities.

Evaluation of Themes for Measurement Development

These themes offer insights that can help to better identify people with disabilities and to advance the measurement of disability generally.

The idea of "doing activities differently" when someone has a health problem or impairment seems very promising. This concept is consistent with the independent living perspective and, importantly, consistent with the definition of disability embodied in the Americans with Disabilities Act (ADA). When the law speaks of a person having a "substantial limitation in a major life activity," such a limitation is defined not in terms of activities the person is unable to engage in, or even has difficulty with, but instead in terms of how the activity is "performed in a manner, duration, or under conditions" that is different from most people (Petrila, 2002).

Thus, the "doing things differently" theme suggests a way of defining disability in terms of specific differences in human behavior that are observed in the context of disability. It is best for constructing good measures that behavioral traits be specific, explicit, and unequivocal. Some examples that would qualify might include using human help or assistive technology to accomplish day to day tasks, or doing such tasks under the supervision of another person. Additional examples would be doing activities using alternate strategies, like doing activities more slowly, or with breaks, or by using different procedures, such as by being tested orally rather than in writing.

This approach can lead to improved accuracy in measuring disability. Because the doing of activities is emphasized, this approach is much more positively oriented than the limitations approach. As a result, people with disabilities may endorse a question about doing things differently when they refrain from endorsing one about being limited in activity, resulting in fewer false negatives.

It is well known that people with disabilities experience problematic social interactions due to stigma, discrimination, avoidance, and so forth. Nevertheless, this may be a difficult construct to use to identify people with disabilities, since characteristics other than disability, including gender, age, ethnicity and race, and sexual orientation are also subject to differential social treatment. It may be difficult to separate out problematic social interactions due to disability from other characteristics a person may have. Nevertheless, the experience of problematic social interactions is quite deeply felt among people with disabilities, and it can be a useful indicator of the social experience of disability.

Management behaviors may involve specific things that people with disabilities may do to ensure better outcomes in their day-to-day lives. Some of these may involve distinct differences between people with and without disabilities in specific behaviors involving planning, prioritizing, and selecting of activities.

People can do things differently when their abilities allow them to function in an environment that is supportive and provides the resources and accommodations that facilitate participation. For some people who do not enjoy a supportive environment, the opportunity to do things differently will not be forthcoming and their activity will be reduced. Despite the clear recognition of the role of the environment in people's day-to-day lives, there is also awareness of the importance of the variability of personal functioning. For some people, personal functioning can be the limiting factor.

A Conceptual Framework

Making use of these concepts, we see disability as an interaction between individual functioning and the environment, in particular the built physical environment and the general social environment, which are often constructed without consideration for the needs of people whose functioning differs from the norm. In such a model, an unaccommodating physical or social environment may result in reduced activity for a person with even a moderate functional limitation. A hostile environment might result in reduced activity for a person with only a slight limitation, while in a benign environment activity may be reduced only for someone with a severe functional limitation.

In this framework, what is clearly important is the impact on a person's activities of limitations in functioning in a particular environment. That impact can occur in various ways: as a different way of performing those activities, such as with assistance or equipment or over a longer period of time; as a need to manage the activities to avoid likely problems in the physical or social environment; as a sense of exclusion or discrimination when performing the activities; or, when functional issues predominate, as an inability to perform some activities, whether necessary or discretionary, at all or to a desired extent.

The approach is consistent with the World Health Organization (2001) International Classification of Functioning, Disability, and Health (ICF), in which disability is seen as arising from a complex interaction among activities engaged in, environmental barriers and facilitators, and aspects of bodily function.

The next step involves the construction of survey questions. We report here our preliminary work toward this aim. Our questions focus on the impact on a person's activities of environmental barriers (problems encountered in the physical and social environment), of environmental facilitators (use of personal assistance and special equipment or assistive technology), and of personal functioning (fatigue, pain, or ill health or the need to do things more slowly).

It is important to recognize that the process of developing a new measure based on new concepts is an evolving one. In this chapter, we present only our initial attempt to develop a new approach to measuring disability. The first step is to develop structured items based on the concepts, then to test their comprehensibility (cognitive testing). Subsequent steps will be to test the items psychometrically in small samples to assess their dimensionality, validity, and reliability.

DAIS: The Disability and Activity Impact Screener (Alpha Version)

Working from the aforementioned themes, we have constructed an initial, alpha version of a new disability measure, the Disability and Activity Impact Screener (DAIS). The DAIS alpha version consists of seven multi-part questions: a condition/impairment screener (Question 0) identifying a broad population with health conditions. impairments. or perceived disabilities, followed by six multi-part disability items (Questions 1–6). These questions focus on ways in which people's activities are impacted by features of the environment (both barriers and facilitators) or by specific aspects of health and functioning. The DAIS incorporates, to a greater or lesser extent, all of the key concepts we identified in our focus group study. In particular, the questions focus primarily on the things people with disabilities do and the ways in which they do them—often differently from other people, either because of or resulting in physical or social barriers—rather than on the things people with disabilities do not or cannot do.

Questions 1 and 2 are about doing things differently, in particular about the use of personal assistance or special equipment. Questions 3 and 4 are about environmental problems, first in the physical environment and then the social environment. Question 5 is again about doing things differently, in particular about taking extra time to do things. Question 6 is about factors relating to personal well-being that may interfere with activities.

Format

Each of the disability items has a two- or three-part format: First, in Part A, a question is asked to identify experiences relevant to the key concept—either a difference from most other people or a problem the respondent has encountered. If the question is answered in the affirmative, then Part B is asked; this question attempts to quantify the impact of the difference or problem on the person's activities. The respondent is offered a list of statements and asked to identify those that apply. The first four items also contain a Part C, asked only of those answering Part A in the negative, aimed at capturing respondents who refrain from engaging in certain activities because either of unmet need or fear of encountering problems. A person would be classified as having a disability if he or she either (1) answers yes to at least one Part A question and also identifies a significant impact in Part B or (2) answers yes to at least one Part C question. It should be emphasized that, while we expect to capture people with all types of disabilities with one or more questions, each question, by itself, is not intended to apply to the entire disability population.

ANNOTATED DAIS QUESTIONNAIRE—ALPHA VERSION

The questionnaire begins with an initial screener question asking about conditions, impairments, and perceived disability. It has two purposes: (1) People who have no significant chronic health condition or impairment and no perceived disability will skip out of the remaining questions, and (2) those identifying themselves as having a health condition, impairment, or perceived disability are asked to specify its source (a condition/impairment list with up to three items), so that information can be referred to in subsequent questions. We believe that naming the condition or impairment in Questions 1–6 will help the respondent focus on aspects relevant to the disability, as opposed to, say, thinking about equipment or technology they use for convenience, rather than in connection with some limitation in functioning.

Question 1 concerns help needed from other people, a key aspect in which people with disabilities do things differently from most other people. One reason that this is a critical issue in the lives of many people with disabilities is that the needed help is not always available, and obtaining adequate, appropriate, and timely assistance can be problematic.

Question 0
Do you have difficulty doing any of these things:
Q 0a. Seeing, hearing, or speaking? Yes/No/DK
Q 0b. Learning, remembering, or getting around? Yes/No/DK

If yes to Q0a or b, ask:
Q 0c. What did you have difficulty with for more than a month, if anything? *Record responses on condition list as "difficulty hearing," "difficulty remembering," etc., or record the specific condition mentioned ("blindness," "cerebral palsy," "Alzheimer's").*

Condition list:
____
____
____

Q 0d. [Other than what you've told me about,] Do you have any physical, mental, or emotional health problems that affect your daily life? Yes/No/DK

If yes to Q0d, ask:
Q 0e. What health problems have you had for more than a month, if any? *Record responses on condition list, above.*

Q 0f. Do you think of yourself as having a disability? Yes/No/DK
Q 0g. Do other people think of you as having a disability? Yes/No/DK

If yes to Q0f or g and condition list is empty, ask:
Q 0h. What condition or specific type of disability do you have? *Record responses on condition list, above, or if no answer, record "disability."*

If no entries on condition list, stop.

This question is a broadening of the traditional questions on activities of daily living (ADL) and instrumental activities of daily living (IADL) to include help from others in mobility or navigation (for example, people with visual impairments), in lifting or carrying, in communicating (such as sign language interpreters) or reading, in keeping track of things (e.g., for a person with a cognitive limitation), or remembering things (cognitive or mental health disability).

Part B identifies four areas of impact that having the needed help enables. Response 1 is meant for people who get assistance with ADLs or other basic personal needs. Response 2 is for those who get help in order to carry out responsibilities related to work (e.g., a job coach, assistant, reader, interpreter), school, the family, or the household. Responses 3 and 4 are for people needing assistance in more discretionary activities, including social and other leisure activities.

Part C, which is asked of people who do not get help, attempts to capture unmet need for help that would have enabled a greater level of participation.

Question 1
Some people with health conditions or limitations get help from other people. They might need help in getting around or finding their way around, lifting or carrying things, communicating, reading, keeping track of things, or remembering things.

Q 1a. As a result of your [condition list], do you get help from other people? Yes/Sometimes/No/DK

If No or DK, skip to Question 1c.

Q 1b. Please tell me whether these statements are true about you:

This help allows you to...

(1) Take care of your personal needs, such as bathing, dressing, or getting around the house. Yes/Sometimes/No
(2) Do other things you need to do, like working, going to school, or doing household or family tasks. Yes/Sometimes/No
(3) Spend more time with friends or family. Yes/Sometimes/No
(4) Do other social or recreational activities for fun. Yes/Sometimes/No
Skip to Q 2.

Q 1c. Are there things you miss out on because you don't get the help you need? Yes/Sometimes/No

Question 2 is about use of assistive technology, another aspect of doing things differently, and one that often entails stigma, because device use can increase the visibility of the impairment. The question is meant to include all types of technology and equipment: mobility devices such as wheelchairs, canes, and walkers; navigation technology such as talking signs; communication devices such as text telephones, telephone amplifiers, speech synthesizers, and screen readers; and devices that remind people to do things or help them locate things.

Parts B and C are nearly identical to Question 1.

Question 3 is about environmental barriers that hinder mobility, navigation, or communication. The question is intended to refer mostly to barriers encountered in the physical environment—barriers in the social environment are primarily addressed in Question 4. Architectural barriers are meant to be included, as are barriers to navigation such as inadequate signage (absence of Braille signs or of signs indicating accessible pathways) and barriers to communication (absence of sign language interpreters, for example).

Because people with disabilities engage in very diverse activities in diverse settings, we have avoided specifying any particular activity or location, but instead ask whether barriers are encountered, presumably in the course of the respondent's normal activities. Part B makes explicit the connection to whatever daily activities the person engages in. The respondent is asked to select from among five statements regarding the impact that such barriers have on these activities:

Question 2
Some people with health conditions or limitations use special equipment or assistive devices. Equipment or devices can help people get around, lift or carry things, see, read, hear, communicate, find things, or remember things.

Q 2a. As a result of your [condition list], do you use any kind of special equipment or assistive devices? Yes/No/DK

If No or DK, skip to Question 2c.

Q 2b. Please tell me whether these statements are true about you:

Special equipment or assistive devices allow you to…

(1) Take care of your personal needs, such as bathing, dressing, or getting around the house. Yes/Sometimes/No
(2) Do other things you need to do, like working, going to school, or doing household or family tasks. Yes/Sometimes/No
(3) Spend more time with friends or family. Yes/Sometimes/No
(4) Do other social or recreational activities for fun. Yes/Sometimes/No
Skip to Q 3.

Q 2c. Are there things you miss out on because you don't have the special equipment or assistive devices you need? Yes/Sometimes/No

Response 1 indicates that barriers interfere with activities, requiring changes in plans. Response 2 is for people who successfully plan ahead so as to avoid those problems; this impact item gets at the management strategies that focus group participants often discussed. Response 3 is the most severe impact, of activities prevented by barriers. Response 4 is for those who feel that they are excluded from participation (i.e., discriminated against) because of barriers.

Part C, asked only of people who do not report encountering physical barriers, is intended to capture people who avoid certain activities, situations, or locations that are known to involve barriers that would hinder their participation.

Question 4 addresses problems in the social environment, a very central theme in the focus group discussions. People often spoke of feeling alienated or excluded as a result of inappropriate treatment by other people, even to the extent of avoiding certain activities or settings because of the way they had been treated in the past. Poor treatment can come from family members, co-workers, salespersons, attendants, or people asked for casual assistance. The problem seems to affect people with all types of disabilities, who may be ignored, patronized, offered unnecessary or excessive help, or asked inappropriate questions. People whose appearance or behavior is out of the ordinary—whether due to a visible physical impairment or disfigurement, use of special equipment or a different means of communication, or a mental health or neurological condition or cognitive impairment—are especially vulnerable.

Question 3
Some people who have health conditions or limitations find that barriers or obstacles make it difficult for them to get into places, move from place to place, find their way around, or communicate with people.

Q 3a. As someone with [condition list], do you come across barriers or obstacles to doing these things? Yes/Sometimes/No/DK

If No or DK, skip to Question 3c.

Q 3b. Please tell me whether these statements are true about you:

When doing your daily activities…

(1) You sometimes have to change your plans because of barriers or obstacles. Yes/No
(2) You sometimes have to plan ahead in order to avoid barriers or obstacles. Yes/No
(3) Barriers or obstacles sometimes stop you from doing the things you want to do. Yes/No
(4) You sometimes feel left out because of barriers or obstacles. Yes/No
Skip to Q 4.

Q 3c. Are there things you miss out on because barriers or obstacles would stop you from doing them? Yes/Sometimes/No

As in Question 3, we are asking the respondent to generalize across whatever activities they typically engage in, whether in public or private, while working, engaging in social activities, shopping, or remaining at home. Note that, in both of these questions, we have intentionally refrained from using the familiar phrasing, "Because of a health condition or impairment...," which requires the person to attribute the problems they encounter to their health or impairment, rather than to the environment. Instead, we ask that the barrier or inappropriate treatment be connected with the health condition or impairment ("As someone with…" in Q. 3 or "As a result of..." in Q. 4).

Part B is very similar to that of Question 3, except that there is an additional item, #1, asking about extra care needed in order to avoid poor treatment (another aspect of management strategies). People who report no poor treatment are asked Part C, which attempts to identify people with hidden conditions or disabilities, who are then asked whether non-disclosure of their condition is a reason for the lack of poor treatment.

Question 5 addresses another way in which people with many disabilities do things differently than most other people—taking more time to accomplish necessary or discretionary activities. In our focus groups, people spoke of the increased length of time it took them to do things—especially basic personal care activities like daily grooming—often resulting in insufficient time left over for other activities. People with mobility impairments may also need longer to travel from place to place, those with speech or hearing impairments may need more time to communicate with others, people with learning or other cognitive disabilities may take longer to read or to absorb information, and people with mental health disabilities may take longer due to issues of motivation or compulsive behavior.

Question 4
Q 4a. As a result of your [condition list], do some people treat you badly or rudely? Yes/Sometimes/No/DK

If No or DK, skip to Question 4c.

Q 4b. Please tell me whether these statements are true about you:

When doing your daily activities…

(1) You have to be extra careful when dealing with people so that they won't treat you badly or rudely. Yes/Sometimes/No
(2) You sometimes have to change your plans because people treat you badly or rudely. Yes/No
(3) You sometimes have to plan ahead in order to avoid being treated badly or rudely. Yes/No
(4) You sometimes miss out on things because people treat you badly or rudely. Yes/No
(5) You sometimes feel left out because people treat you badly or rudely. Yes/No
Skip to Q 5.

Q 4c.
(1) Is that because most people don't know about your [condition list]? Yes/No/DK

If yes, ask:
(2) If people knew about your [condition list], would they treat you badly or rudely? Yes/Sometimes/No

Question 5
Some people with health conditions or limitations take more time than most other people to do things. For example, they might take more time to get around, take care of their personal needs, communicate, read, or learn.

Q 5a. As a result of your [condition list], do you take more time to do things? Yes/Sometimes/No/DK

If No or DK, skip to Question 6.

Q 5b. Thinking about the things you take more time to do, please tell me whether these statements are true about you:

(1) You do those things less completely than you would like. Yes/Sometimes/No
(2) You avoid doing those things. Yes/Sometimes/No
(3) Because it takes you more time to do certain things, you have less time for other activities that are important to you. Yes/Sometimes/No

The five responses in Part B identify the impact that taking more time has on daily activities. Those endorsing Response 1 are unable to fulfill all their personal needs. Response 2 is for those unable to complete all their major responsibilities, such as work, schoolwork, or household tasks. Responses 3 and 4 are for those unable to participate fully in social and leisure activities. Response 5 gets at a management strategy that the focus group participants often mentioned, of having to prioritize activities and attempt only the most important.

Question 6 addresses additional aspects of the experience of disability that relate more directly to individual rather than environmental causes. Some focus group participants speak of not being able to participate in activities due to poor mental or physical health, to lack of energy or stamina, or to chronic pain. The extent of these problems often varies from day to day, meaning that they are uncertain of their ability to participate in future activities, making longer term planning (for example, committing to returning to work) difficult or impossible.

Part B is similar to that in Question 5.

Question 6
a. As a result of your [condition list], are you often tired, weak, sick, or in pain? Yes/Sometimes/No/DK

If No or DK, skip to end.

b. Please tell me whether these statements are true about you:

Because of this problem…

(1) There are days when you skip taking care of some of your personal needs, such as bathing, dressing, or grooming. Yes/Sometimes/No
(2) There are days when you skip doing other things you need to do, like working, going to school, or doing household or family tasks. Yes/Sometimes/No
(3) There are days when you skip social or recreational activities for fun. Yes/Sometimes/No

Further Development and Testing of the DAIS Questionnaire

A previous version of this chapter was circulated among experts in both survey development and conceptualizations of disability. At the same time, the questions were cognitively tested in individual interviews with people with disabilities, at UCSF and in the Cognitive Laboratory at the National Center for Health Statistics. The questionnaire was revised based on feedback from these sources. A second round of cognitive testing was undertaken at UCSF. Minor revisions occurred following that test. People with disabilities generally reacted quite favorably to these questions, in contrast to negative appraisals of standard activity limitation questions.

The lack of detail in the questions is intentional,because the purpose of the questionnaire is to identify people with disabilities concisely. The next step will be to collect sample data, conduct validity testing, and compare the DAIS responses with those to other, more familiar disability measures, and assess their reliability and validity. We are planning on testing these questions in subsamples of ongoing surveys.

As part of the validity testing, we will also be comparing responses to the individual questions against one another. The aim is to be able to identify those questions and impact items that are most effective in discriminating between people with and without disabilities, and to be able to reduce the questionnaire down to a short-form version that could be included in general-purpose, national surveys to identify people with disabilities.

Conclusion

Based on focus group discussions with people with disabilities about their lived experience, new concepts emerged with promise for improving survey measures about people with disabilities. These concepts generally are concerned with how people with disabilities perform activities differently from other people, and the personal (management strategies) and environmental conditions (barriers and facilitators) that allow or prevent that from occurring. The development of the DAIS, and highly favorable responses obtained from cognitive testing with people with disabilities, provide an example of how qualitative measurement discovery can help to achieve the goal of improving the relevance of survey items to people with disabilities and their experiences.

REFERENCES

Altman, B. M. (2001). Disability definitions, models, classification schemes, and applications. In G. L. Albrecht, K. D. Seelman and M. Bury (Eds.), *Handbook of Disability Studies* (pp. 97-122). Thousand Oaks, CA, US: Sage Publications, Inc.

Bickenbach, J. E., Chatterji, S., Bradley, E. M., and Ustun, T. B. (1999). Models of disablement, universalism and the international classification of impairments, disabilities and handicaps. *Social Science and Medicine, 48,* 1173-1187.

Commission on Chronic Illness. 1957. Chronic Illness in the United States. Vol. 4, Chronic Illness in a Large City. Cambridge, Mass.: Harvard University Press.

Fougeyrollas, P., and Beauregard, L. (2001). Disability: An interactive person-environment social creation. In G. L. Albrecht, K. D. Seelman and M. Bury (Eds.), *Handbook of Disability Studies* (pp. 171-194). Thousand Oaks, CA: Sage.

Fujiura, G. T. and Rutkowski-Kmitta, V. (2001). Counting disability. In G. L. Albrecht, K. D. Seelman and M. Bury (Eds.*), Handbook of Disability Studies* (pp. 69-96). Thousand Oaks, CA: Sage.

Gill, C. J. (2001). Divided understandings: The social experience of disability. In G. L. Albrecht, K. D. Seelman and M. Bury (Eds.), *Handbook of Disability Studies* (pp. 351-372). Thousand Oaks, CA, US: Sage Publications, Inc.

Glaser, B. G. and Strauss, A. L. (1967). *The Discovery of Grounded Theory: Strategies for Qualitative Research*. Chicago: Aldine Pub. Co.

Gray, D. B. and Hendershot, G. E. (2000). The ICIDH-2: Developments for a new era of outcomes research. *Archives of Physical Medicine and Rehabilitation, 81*(12 Suppl 2), S10-14.

Hahn, H. and Hegamin, A. P. (2001). Assessing scientific measures of disability. *Journal of Disability Policy Studies, 12*(2), 114-121.

Kitzinger, J. (1994). The methodology of focus groups: the importance of interaction between research participants. *Sociology of Health and Illness, 16*(1), 103-121.

McHorney, CA. (2003). Ten recommendations ofr advancing patient-centered outcomes measurement for older persons. *Ann Intern Med* 139:403-409.

McNeil, J. (2001) "Americans with Disabilities, 1997." *Current Population Reports* No. P70-73. Washington, D.C. U.S. Department of the Census.

Meyers, A. R. and Andresen, E. M. (2000). Enabling our instruments: Accommodation, universal design, and access to participation in research. *Archives of Physical Medicine and Rehabilitation, 81(*12 Suppl 2), S5-9.

Morgan, D. L. (1997). *Focus Groups as Qualitative Research (2nd ed.).* Thousand Oaks, CA, US: Sage Publications, Inc.

O'Day, B. and Killeen, M. (2002). Research on the lives of persons with disabilities: the emerging importance of qualitative research methodologies. *Journal of Disability Policy Studies, 13*(1), 9-15.

Petrila, J. (2002). The U.S. Supreme Court Narrows the Definition of Disability Under the Americans With Disabilities Act. *Law and Psychiatry, 53* (7): 797-798, 801.

Scotch, R. K. and Schriner, K. (1997). Disability as human variation: Implications for policy. *Annals of the American Academy of Political and Social Science* , 549(Jan), 148-159.

Stern, S. (2003). Counting people with disabilities: how survey methodology influences estimates in Census 2000 and the Census 2000 Supplementary Survey. Washington: US Census Bureau. *http://www.census.gov/hhes/www/disability/finalstern.pdf*

Stern, S. and Brault, M. (2005). Disability data from the American Community Survey: a brief examination of the effects of a question redesign in 2003. Washington: US Census Bureau. *http://www.census.gov/hhes/www/disability/ACS_disability.pdf*

Stewart, A. L. and Napoles-Springer, A. (2000). Health-related quality-of-life assessments in diverse population groups in the United States. *Medical Care, 38*(Suppl9), II102-II124.

US Department of Labor. (2005). Delivering on the Promise: U.S. Department of Labor

Self-Evaluation to Promote Community Living for People with Disabilities Report to the President On Executive Order 13217. Washington: US DOL. Accessed June 24, 2005. http://www.hhs.gov/newfreedom/final/pdf/dol.pdf

World Health Organization. (2001). The International Classification of Functioning, Disability, and Health-ICF. Geneva: WHO. iii+299 pages ISBN 91 4 154542 9.

In: Towards Best Practices for Surveying People..., Volume 1 ISBN 1-60021-195-X
Editors: Thilo Kroll, David Keer et al., pp. 165-179

Chapter 10

A MULTI-MODE APPROACH FOR SURVEYING VISUALLY IMPAIRED POPULATIONS

Patrick Murray[1]
Monmouth University Polling Institute
400 Cedar Avenue
West Long Branch, NJ 07764

The author wishes to thank the *New Jersey Commission for the Blind and Visually Impaired* for allowing these data to be used for public research and education and two anonymous reviewers for their helpful comments.

ABSTRACT

This case study examines the efficacy of conducting a self-administered survey with a visually impaired population. The study was conducted with clients of the Vocational Rehabilitation Program at the New Jersey Commission for the Blind and Visually Impaired. The basic design was multi-modal, involving a mailed survey packet with options for completing the survey in four self-administered formats (in writing on a large-print document, by Braille, computer disk, or audio tape) and one interview-assisted mode (by contacting a staffed toll-free telephone line). A follow-up survey was conducted with a sample of non-participants to assess reasons for non-response. The study was later replicated. The study found that less expensive self-administered modes can be used to conduct valid probability surveys with a visually impaired population. However, it may be important that an interviewer-assisted mode be available, if not for the final survey results to be representative of the full population, then to fulfill other accessibility obligations.

[1] (732) 263-5858, Fax: (732) 263-5859, pdmurray@monmouth.edu

INTRODUCTION

Surveying people with disabilities is a demanding but important challenge. Options for modes of interviewing are limited, particularly when the population in question has visual impairments. Federally-funded vocational rehabilitation ("VR") programs are required to conduct a triennial consumer satisfaction assessment as a condition of their funding. The federal guidelines are ambiguous on how such an assessment is to be conducted. Those charged with conducting statistically rigorous evaluations of visually impaired individuals on very limited resources run up against countless problems. In many cases, VR programs gather information in a less than methodologically sound manner. Evaluations are conducted with convenience samples or with a very limited number of program participants. Some believe that, without an exhaustive and expensive set of survey modes, it is not possible to conduct a true probability survey that can be drawn to reflect – or "generalize to" – the experiences and opinions of the larger population.

In 1997, the New Jersey Commission for the Blind and Visually Impaired contracted with researchers at Rutgers University to conduct a consumer[2] survey using a comprehensive survey methodology in order to fulfill this requirement. The nature of this population's disability – vocational rehabilitation program participants who were visually impaired – posed some unique methodological issues. The population for the initial survey was comprised of all VR consumers whose case was either closed during the previous fiscal year or in an open active status as of the close of the prior fiscal year. The challenge was to conduct a survey with enough individuals that would accurately reflect the views of all individuals covered in that population.

Many, if not most, surveys with visually impaired individuals occur on a very small scale or with individuals who are currently active in a program (Craven, Crudden and McBroom, Golledge and Marston). Some large scale general population surveys of people with disabilities obviously include individuals with visual impairments. However, this chapter is concerned with surveys conducted specifically to assess services related to visual disabilities. In general practice, the methodologies used to conduct visual impairment population surveys include individuals who are relatively easy to contact and do not require extensive resources for data collection. In these instances, the sampled individuals may be more motivated to participate by virtue of the fact that they are currently receiving some direct benefit.

While the population for the current study was relatively small (N=1432) in general population survey terms, it was still larger than that found in the typical disability program assessment. Moreover, these individuals were spread throughout the state of New Jersey. Many in the sample had left the program and thus there was no easy way to "intercept" them for the survey (e.g. interviews conducted as they attended a service or program). In studies of very small populations, a one-on-one approach would provide the optimal response. However, the total number of potential participants and the geographic distances for this population made personal interviews unfeasible.

Another option for this type of research is to embark on a telephone survey. Unfortunately, full and complete telephone information was not available for all consumers at the time the initial survey was developed. Therefore any telephone sample drawn from this population may have been skewed.

---

[2] The word "consumer" is used here to denote clients of the vocational rehabilitation program.

The crux of the problem in deciding which modes of interviewing are acceptable and which are not lies in the definition of visual impairment. If a large number of program participants are totally blind, a self administered survey would not be practicable. However, in the vocational rehabilitation population, the definition of a visual impairment runs a very large gamut of visual acuity. In this case, client information available from the VR program indicated that a majority of consumers would be able to read a large print document and may even prefer to complete the questionnaire on their own. As such, the research team endeavored to design a study protocol based on a standard self-administered mail format, supplemented by alternate modes of access.[3] The results of this study showed that some modes were more useful than others in boosting the response rate. However, no single mode significantly affected the substantive results of the survey itself.

I. METHODS

The original survey was conducted in 1997. The research team was provided with a list of 1432 consumers who met the study population parameters. This included all currently active clients whose case was past the "assessment" stage and any client whose case was closed (either successfully or unsuccessfully in rehab terms) during the prior fiscal year. This population was reduced to 1266 after the list was cleaned for clients who were deceased or had ended services because they moved out of state. Because of the small population size, the research team chose to include all 1266 consumers in the study.

The questionnaire itself was pre-tested with a small group of current VR consumers who had visual impairments but were able to read large print documents. The consumers were asked about the survey content as well as their preferences for format. Based on their recommendations the questionnaire was printed in a 15-point standard Times Roman serif font. This recommendation ran counter to the standard practice for producing large print documents. Much of the literature on large print specifications suggests that large print documents should be printed in a 16 to 18 point font. Also, many of these sources recommend a sans serif font, such as Arial (for example, see Braille Plus, CPS, Kitchel, Roundtable, Washington). However, survey questionnaires are laid out in a much different manner than a standard written text document. A survey instrument has larger white spaces and more visual cues (such as dot leaders) that may heighten reading access. These assumptions were not tested further, but the research team decided to go with the recommendations of the pre-test group.

The basic methodology of the survey followed a standard mail three-wave design (Dillman). This design involves a full mailing of all materials, followed by a large-print reminder card or letter approximately 7 days after the initial mailing, and then a second full survey packet about 10 days after the reminder mailing. The survey packet included a 12-page large print questionnaire booklet, a postage paid reply envelope, and a cover letter from the director of the New Jersey Commission for the Blind and Visually Impaired.

[3] Some recent research has discussed the potential offered by Internet access among people with visual impairments (e.g. Gerber and Kirchner). While access and functionality of this mode is improving, it is still limited. Thus it is difficult to construct a representative probability sample of nearly any population using this mode as a survey research data collection tool.

The cover letter was provided in both large print and Brailled format for all packets. In addition to introducing the study, the cover letter included information about completing the survey in alternate formats. These formats included receiving the questionnaire in Braille, on computer disk, or read on audio tape. A toll-free telephone number was given for respondents to contact the research team. This telephone line was staffed by an interviewer from 10:00 am to 8:00 pm Monday through Friday for a period of four weeks. The cover letter indicated that respondents could also choose to complete the interview over the phone during these times. During times when the telephone line was not staffed, voice mail was available to take messages on the toll-free number.

Seven days following the initial mailing, reminder postcards were sent to all who had not responded. Another full survey packet was mailed to non-respondents 10 days after the reminder mailing. The research team filled requests for 5 copies of the questionnaire in Braille, 2 on audio tape, and 2 on computer disk. Of these, three Braille surveys were returned (with the responses circled in pencil) and one computer disk was returned (with an 'X' or other answer typed in the computer document). A total of 377 large print surveys were returned and 144 interviews were completed over the telephone.

Table 1. Key Differences In Research Modes For 1997 And 2003 Surveys

	Available	
	1997	2003
Survey packet		
--Large print cover letter	X	X
--Brailled cover letter	X	X
--Large print questionnaire	X	X
--Postage paid reply envelope	X	X
Reminder postcard		
--Large print	X	X
Alternate self-administered modes available upon respondent request		
--Braille questionnaire	X	
--Text file on computer disk	X	
--Survey read on audio tape	X	
Interviewer-assisted telephone mode		
--Toll-free line staffed during weekdays	X	
--Toll-free voice mail available during unstaffed hours for interviewers to return calls	X	X

This study was replicated in 2003, utilizing the exact same questionnaire. In this case, the population included 1477 VR clients. Resources for the more recent survey were reduced in real terms relative to the 1997 survey. While the same survey instrument was used and three-wave mail design was utilized (including a Brailled cover letter), the number of alternative formats was limited. The 2003 survey did not offer the questionnaire in Braille, audio tape or computer disk. Also, while a toll-free number was provided, it was not staffed as in the initial study. Callers were directed into a voice mail system, which was checked regularly. Calls were returned by a trained interviewer. This substantially reduced the cost involved in the survey process. Key differences in mode availability for both studies are summarized in Table 1. In the end, a total of 528 large print surveys were returned and 65 interviews were completed over the telephone for the 2003 survey.

Conducting the survey by mail only would have produced a response rate of 30-31 percent in either year.[4] The staffed interviewer-assisted telephone option boosted the response rate by another 11 percentage points in 1997. The other available modes (Braille, computer disk, and audio tape) had no impact on the response rate. In 2003, the toll-free voice mail system boosted the response rate by another 5 percent. Therefore, the key issue was whether including an interviewer-assisted mode improves the representativeness of mail survey results for a consumer satisfaction study with visually impaired individuals, and if so, whether it is necessary to provide a staffed telephone line. The following section of this chapter first examines the results of the 1997 survey and then follows with a comparative discussion of the 2003 survey.

SURVEY RESULTS

Assessing the soundness of the original 1997 survey results hinges on two points of comparison. The first point is whether the survey participants "look like" the entire population of VR clients. The second point is whether the respondents who participated by self-administered mode "look like" those who participated by interviewer-assisted mode.

Reading Mode

Since accessibility is the prime concern, the first area of examination is the means of access that this population can physically use – in this case, their available reading mode. When visually impaired consumers enter the New Jersey VR program, they are asked for their preferred mode of receiving written materials. This information is updated throughout the course of a consumer's tenure with the VR program. Table 2 presents the distribution of preferred reading modes among all clients, clients who participated in the survey, and clients who did not participate.

Overall, the pool of those who participated in the survey looks very much like the total VR population in terms of reading mode. Those who read regular or large print are somewhat more likely to have participated by mail than by telephone. However, the differences in marginal distributions are not that sizable. Comparing the VR population to just the subgroup of mail respondents shows similar levels of print readers (65% to 67%), Braille readers (7% to 6%), and audio tape users (15% to 14%). Utilizing a chi square test finds no statistically significant difference between the reading modes of survey participants and non-participants. More importantly, there is no statistically significant difference in the reading mode preferences for mail participants compared to phone participants.

[4] This response rate is similar to other large-scale surveys of visually impaired populations. For example, see Eggett.

Even though these differences are not statistically significant, there are some issues worth noting. Print readers make up 67 percent of mail respondents and 54 percent of telephone respondents. Clearly, the large-print questionnaire was adequate for many VR consumers who can read print. Yet a sizable number in this group still felt more comfortable completing the survey with an interviewer.

Table 2. 1997 Survey Participation By Reading Mode*

	VR population (n=1266)	All participants (n=525)	*Participated by mail (n=377)*	*Participated by phone (n=144)*	Did not partici-pate (n=741)
Reading Mode					
-- Unknown	9%	10%	*9%*	*13%*	9%
-- Regular print	29	26	*28*	*22*	30
-- Large print	36	37	*39*	*32*	35
-- Braille	7	8	*6*	*12*	6
-- Tapes	15	14	*14*	*17*	16
-- CCTV	3	3	*2*	*3*	2
-- Non-reader	2	2	*2*	*2*	3

* *Determined from NJCBVI case records.*

	Participants v. Non-participants	Mail v. Phone Participants
Chi-Square analysis	p=.439	p=.127

At the same time, 20 percent of those who participated using the large print survey were designated as Braille or audiotape "readers." This compares to 29 percent of telephone participants. Keep in mind that only 4 (out 525) survey participants chose to utilize the Braille, computer disk, or audiotape modes to respond. Thus, it seems that a combination of large print and telephone modes provides an adequate level of access for alternate reading mode consumers.

The survey's response rate was not altered by the availability of alternate self-administered modes. When given the choice, survey participants who had earlier expressed a preference for receiving materials in Braille, computer disk or audio tape decided chose to complete the survey using the large-print questionnaire or telephone option. Since only 4 individuals used one of the alternate self-administered modes, it is not possible to make any statistical statements about how they differed from other study participants. Therefore, this chapter, of necessity, focuses on the key difference of large-print mail versus interviewer assisted telephone modes.

Demographic Characteristics

Another set of comparisons can be made with the demographic characteristics of survey participants. Table 3 illustrates the distributions for gender, race, region of the state, corrected visual acuity, presence of multiple disabilities (other than visual), status of the consumer's VR case, and work status when the consumer's case was first assigned to the VR program.

These demographics are of the type that may be expected to have the greatest impact on survey response. Some (such as gender and race) are applicable to all surveys. The general trend in self-administered surveys (not just those with disability populations) is that men and racial/ethnic minorities are less likely to participate. Furthermore, one may expect residents of urban areas to be less inclined to participate.

Other issues apply more specifically to a survey population with disabilities. These include the severity of visual impairment, the presence of other disabilities which may inhibit survey participation as well as one's working status. Also, case status is included since those for whom VR services are more or less successful may have a different likelihood to participate in a survey about the program.

Table 3. 1997 Profile Of Survey Participants

	VR population (n=1266)	All participants (n=525)*	*Participated by mail (n=377)*	*Participated by phone (n=144)*	Did not participate (n=741)
Gender					
-- Male	51%	48%	*51%*	*40%*	54%
-- Female	49	52	*49*	*60*	46
Race					
-- White	68	73	*77*	*63*	64
-- Black	21	17	*15*	*25*	24
-- Hispanic	11	10	*8*	*12*	12
Region of State					
-- Urban Northeast	19	19	*16*	*26*	19
-- Rural Northwest	22	22	*22*	*21*	22
-- Suburban Shore	17	19	*22*	*11*	16
-- Central Suburbs	23	22	*21*	*26*	23
-- Southern Cities & Towns	19	18	*19*	*16*	20
Corrected Visual Acuity					
-- 20/20 to 20/50	18	17	*16*	*19*	19
-- 20/60 to 20/100	21	19	*21*	*14*	22
-- 20/110 to 20/200	24	27	*29*	*22*	22
-- 20/210 to 20/800	14	11	*10*	*14*	16
-- Some light perception	16	16	*15*	*18*	15
-- Totally blind	8	10	*9*	*14*	6
Multiple Disabilities					
-- Yes	38	38	*38*	*41*	38
VR Case Status					
-- Open/Counseling	6	6	*6*	*7*	6
-- Open/Training	29	34	*32*	*37*	25
-- Open/Ready or Employed	12	12	*13*	*11*	12
-- Closed/Successful	33	33	*34*	*31*	32
-- Closed/Unsuccessful	11	7	*7*	*6*	14
-- Post-Employment	10	9	*9*	*8*	11
Work Status at Assignment					
-- Employed	26	27	*29*	*24*	25
-- Student	18	18	*19*	*17*	17
-- Not employed	56	54	*52*	*59*	57

* Includes 377 who completed the survey by mail, 144 by phone and 4 by Braille/computer disk.

Another way to examine the impact of research design on sample representativeness is to look at the "fit" along the marginal distributions for key demographic groups.

Table 3 presents 7 demographic variables with 25 dimensions for comparison (treating gender as a single dimension since it is dichotomous). The difference in distributions between all survey participants (combining mail and telephone responses) and the total VR population is within 3 percentage points on 21 of the 25 dimensions. This is within the basic "margin of error" calculation for a probability sample of this size. The other 4 dimensions in the survey sample are within 5 percentage points of the actual population parameter.

On the face of it, the demographic results indicate that the survey sample (including both mail and telephone respondents) is fairly representative of the population. Would a survey conducted by mail alone have produced a similarly representative sample? Specifically, did the inclusion of an interview-assisted mode improve the representativeness of the total survey sample? At first glance, there seems to have been a slight improvement because of the telephone mode. Inclusion of the telephone mode "helped" improve the marginals on 15 of the 25 demographic dimensions. This means that the overall marginal percentages when comparing mail participants only to mail and phone participants combined moved the entire sample closer to the VR population distribution percentages. For example, after including telephone participants, the distribution of white respondents in the survey sample decreased from 77 percent in the mail only sample to 73 percent for the total sample. This placed the sample distribution 4 percentage points closer to distribution of white consumers found in the VR population (68%).

On the other hand, the telephone survey "hurt" the demographic distributions of the survey along 7 dimensions. The most notable instance of this is gender. Men made up 51 percent of mail survey participants, which matched the gender distribution of the full VR population. However, men were under-represented in the telephone mode and thus skewed the gender distribution for the total sample to 48 percent male.

Of course, the important question is whether any of these differences are statistically significant. The first step of this comparison is between mail and phone participants. Of the 7 main demographic variables tested, there are statistically significant differences for 3 variables when comparing participants by mode. As Table 4 shows, the chi-square value is significant for gender, race, and region. These are three variables where one would expect to find disparities in survey participation by mode among any type of population survey, not just one among people with disabilities.[5]

However, the results also show that there are no statistically significant differences between mail and telephone respondents for the disability-related variables. These are variables one may hypothesize to have a substantial impact on mode of response (i.e. visual acuity, presence of multiple disabilities, VR case status, and work status).

Finding few response difference between the mail and telephone samples does not necessarily mean that the total sample is representative of the population. Chi square analysis shows that there are significant differences between those who participated in the survey (by any mode) and those who did not for 4 of the 7 demographic variables. These include gender, race, visual acuity, and VR case status. There were no statistically significant differences between participants and non-participants on presence of multiple disabilities, work status,

[5] The samples found in general population telephone surveys frequently over-represent women, whites, and suburban residents if no sample selection or demographic quotas are utilized.

and region. In fact, it appears that the inclusion of the telephone assisted mode helped to bring the lower-income urban regional representation into line with the full population distribution.

Table 4. 1997 Profile of Survey Participants

Chi-Square analysis	Participants v. Non-participants	Mail v. Phone Participants
Gender	p=.045	p=.034
Race	p=.003	p=.007
Region of State	p=.692	p=.007
Corrected Visual Acuity	p=.003	p=.075
Multiple Disabilities	p=.934	p=.488
VR Case Status	p=.000	p=.871
Work Status at Assignment	p=.556	p=.337

Among those 4 variables which showed a statistically significant impact on participation, the inclusion of a telephone mode skewed the gender distribution away from the full VR population but pulled the race distribution closer to the population parameter (although still not enough to bring the survey sample fully in line with the VR population distribution on that demographic).

The differences in visual acuity between sample and population distributions are mainly attributable to two adjoining categories – those whose vision is between 20/110 and 20/200 and those whose vision is between 20/210 and 20/800. The 20/110-200 category is slightly over-represented in the survey sample, while the 20/210-800 category is slightly underrepresented.

The differences in VR status are even more telling. For 5 out of 7 categories listed under VR status, the marginal differences between survey participants and the full VR population is no more than a single percentage point. The 2 remaining categories show larger differences: those consumers whose case was active and receiving training were somewhat over-represented in the survey sample, while those whose case was closed unsuccessfully were somewhat under-represented. These are the subgroups who would be expected to have very different levels of satisfaction with VR services. The next section discusses the impact on actual survey findings.

Survey Results

Perhaps the most important issue in any study of public opinion is whether and how the data collection methodology affects the substantive results of the survey. The final data in this study were weighted to correct for disparities in gender, race and VR status between the survey sample and total VR population. Fifteen key variables from the survey were selected and coded into positive, negative and neutral responses. Comparing the weighted data with the unweighted data showed no more than a single percentage point change in any of the marginal distributions across the 15 key survey questions after the data were adjusted. For practical purposes, the unweighted data would have told the same "story" as the weighted data. That is to say, the difference between saying that 75 percent of the VR population feels positively toward the program and saying that number is 74 or 73 percent is substantively inconsequential.

The next question is whether the addition of the telephone mode had a significant impact on the findings of the survey. The unweighted survey results for mail participants and telephone participants are presented in Table 5.

Table 5. 1997 Survey Results By Interview Mode

Affirmative responses	Participated by mail (n=377)	Participated by phone (n=144)	*Differ-ence*	*Chi-Square*
Vocational services were good	36%	28%	*8*	*.059*
Have benefited from services	77	82	*5*	*.063*
Quality of information was good	56	55	*1*	*.182*
Able to choose own vocational goal	72	73	*1*	*.193*
More independent because of program	67	69	*2*	*.222*
Case was closed too soon	35	28	*7*	*.244*
Would recommend CBVI to friends	85	91	*6*	*.250**
Materials given in preferred format	76	75	*1*	*.252*
Did not receive a requested service	30	35	*5*	*.302*
Counselor guidance was good	65	60	*5*	*.376*
Experienced delays in receiving service	40	44	*4*	*.410*
Only now know of other services	22	25	*3*	*.493*
Length of waiting time was good	55	62	*7*	*.767*
Overall experience was good	68	73	*5*	*.834*
Rights were clearly explained	76	72	*4*	*.873*

* *Chi-square value not reliable*

As Table 5 shows, the difference in positive responses between the two sample modes ranges from 1 to 8 percentage points for 15 key items in the survey. However, the chi-square value was not significant for any of these items. Therefore, one cannot conclude that the views of visually impaired consumers who completed a self-administered questionnaire were significantly different from those who utilized an interviewer-assisted mode.

Furthermore, the marginal effect of the two modes is not predictable. The mail sample tended to be more positive than the telephone sample in their assessments on 8 of the 15 items, while the telephone sample gave more positive responses than the mail sample on the remaining 7.

While this analysis indicates that the two modes made no significant impact on the substantive survey results, it is important to note that all these survey participants were self-selected to some degree. Despite the fact that the survey sample demographics were relatively close to the full population, the research team wanted to assess whether there were any accessibility-related issues among those who did not participate. To this end, 70 non-participating consumers with listed telephone numbers were randomly selected and contacted via phone to ascertain their reasons for not responding to the survey.

More than half of these non-respondents said they received the survey but chose not to participate. The main reasons for this were either they did not have the time or they felt the survey did not apply to them. These rationales are typical reasons for non-response in any public opinion survey. About 10 percent of non-respondents claimed that they had in fact returned the survey. It may be likely that this claim arose out of social desirability – specifically, the desire to appear as a willing participant when confronted.

About 1-in-4 did not recall receiving the survey. Anecdotal evidence from the information offered by these non-responders suggests that some people with visual impairments rely on others to open and sort their mail. It is not clear how many of these consumers would not have been told about the survey (which is an interesting question for a separate study). Another 5 percent said that they needed to receive the information in another format. While this may have affected some individuals' ability to participate, the number of consumers who did not participate due to non-voluntary reasons is small. Even if they had participated, the overall impact on the survey results would have most likely been too small to change the findings. This conclusion is based on a comparison of the survey responses given by initial non-responders with data from the original sample.

2003 Survey Comparison

Now, the next question – and a particularly important one when resources are tight – is whether providing a staffed toll-free telephone line is necessary to achieve valid results. As mentioned earlier in this chapter, the 1997 study was replicated in 2003. The latter study used the same sampling methodology and survey instrument, but provided a toll-free voice mail line rather than an interviewer-staffed telephone line. The 1997 and 2003 surveys had similar response rates for the self-administered mail portion of survey. However, the interviewer-assisted telephone response in 2003 was half that of the 1997 survey.

As Table 6 shows, the distribution of preferred reading modes in 2003 is similar to that of the client population in 1997. Those preferring large print are somewhat more numerous in 2003, but the overall distributions are comparable. As in 1997, there was no significant difference between the final survey sample and the full population along this important accessibility characteristic. There do appear to be some differences between the mail and telephone participants, but these are parallel to the differences found in the 1997 survey and work to contribute to the overall representativeness of the final survey sample.

As with the 1997 data, comparisons were made between the 2003 survey sample and the full consumer population for 7 demographic variables along 25 dimensions. While it is true that 4 of the 7 main demographic groups are statistically significant – as they were with the 1997 data – these differences are substantively minor (see Table 7). Specifically, 19 of 25 dimensions in the sample fell within the margin of error (3 percentage points of the population) for the 2003 survey. The remaining 6 items were within 4 percentage points of the population parameter. Furthermore, there was only one statistically significant difference (for visual acuity) between mail and telephone participants among these 7 demographic variables.

2003 responses to the same 15 survey questions from 1997 were also examined for differences between mail and telephone participants. Only one of these ("vocational services were good") was statistically significant at the $p<.05$ level. However, due to small cell sizes in the 2003 survey for telephone participants, the chi-square test could only be reliably run on 6 of the 15 items. More indicative of any modal bias may be the actual marginal differences between the mail and telephone participants. In most cases (12 of 15), the actual percentage point difference on any survey item was 6 points or fewer. Two items had differences of about 10 percentage points ("materials given in preferred format" and "did not receive a requested service") and one item had a truly significant difference of 22 percentage points ("case was closed too soon") between mail and telephone participants.

Table 6. 2003 Survey Participation By Reading Mode*

	VR population (n=1477)	All participants (n=528)	*Participated by mail (n=463)*	*Participated by phone (n=65)*	Did not participate (n=949)
Reading Mode					
-- Unknown	10%	8%	*8%*	*6%*	11%
-- Regular print	24	23	*23*	*22*	25
-- Large print	44	47	*49*	*37*	42
-- Braille	6	6	*5*	*14*	6
-- Tapes	12	12	*11*	*18*	13
-- CCTV	3	3	*3*	*3*	2
-- Non-reader	1	1	*1*	*0*	1

* *Determined from NJCBVI case records.*

	Participants v. Non-participants	Mail v. Phone Participants
Chi-Square analysis	p=.274	p=.037*

* *Chi-square value not reliable*

Table 7. 2003 Profile Of Survey Participants

Chi-Square analysis	Participants v. Non-participants	Mail v. Phone Participants
Gender	p=.238	p=.670
Race	p=.036	p=.154
Region of State	p=.279	p=.090
Corrected Visual Acuity	p=.009	p=.001
Multiple Disabilities	p=.766	p=.632
VR Case Status	p=.001	p=.563
Work Status at Assignment	p=.030	p=.182

CONCLUSIONS

The importance of accessibility when conducting a survey of people with disabilities should not be understated, especially when the disability is vision-related and the preferred survey mode is self-administered. However, the experience of this study showed that an "inclusive" methodology does not necessarily mean that every conceivable type of access needs to be provided in order to achieve valid survey results.

Few Braille readers and audio tape users requested those particular types of accommodations in the 1997 survey. In fact, even if the survey had only provided for a self-administered mail format, the final sample would have been proportionally representative of all reading modes.

The inclusion of an interviewer-assisted telephone mode did affect the demographic distributions of the sample somewhat. For instance, women were more likely to participate by telephone. The mail sample in 1997 over-represented white consumers, while the telephone sample was closer in representation for race/ethnicity in this particular population. This mode effect was less evident in the 2003 survey.

Consumers with multiple disabilities participated in the survey in proportion to their segment of the client population and were just as likely to use either survey mode. In terms of corrected visual acuity, those whose vision was between 20/60 and 20/200 were more likely to participate by mail than by telephone. In comparison, consumers whose vision was worse than 20/200 were more likely to use the telephone mode. The only group who was significantly under-represented in both the mail and telephone samples were those with closed cases following an unsuccessful rehabilitation. However, these differences were relatively minor.

Furthermore, the survey results indicate that the inclusion of an interviewer-assisted mode or other alternatives is not in and of itself necessary to produce statistically representative survey results. However, when conducting a survey of this nature, it may be important to include alternatives to enhance the face validity of the results. If nothing else, making a good faith effort to provide greater access when conducting disability-related surveys is the right thing to do.

These results seem to indicate that a truly representative survey of a "visually impaired" population can be conducted with limited resources. This particular study found that some "preferred" reading modes (i.e. Braille, audio tape, computer disk) were in fact shunned by consumers in favor of either a standard large-print self-administered format or a telephone interview. This is an important finding for programs and agencies that have shied away from conducting methodologically rigorous evaluations because of concerns over the resources needed for such an endeavor. The 2003 results also show that providing a full-time interview staff to receive incoming calls may not be critical to fielding a valid survey. Even in 1997, many of the telephone interviews were in fact conducted in response to messages that were left during times of day when the phone was not staffed. It appears that providing a toll-free voice mail box to leave a message and number for an interviewer to call back may result in a lower overall response rate for the survey, but may provide an adequate alternative when resources are limited.

In sum, the initial response rate for the self-administered mail survey produced a 30 to 31 percent response rate in both years that the survey was conducted. The addition of a toll-free telephone option increased the response rate by 5 or 11 percentage points depending on whether the telephone line was staffed. The addition of self-administered modes other than large-print (i.e. Braille, computer disk, or audio tape) did not improve the survey's response rate or representativeness. Researchers who are concerned with the overall response rate of their surveys could boost participation (and representativeness) by selecting a secondary sample of non-responders to contact by telephone after the initial field period has ended.

The findings presented in this chapter indicate that it is possible to conduct a valid self-administered mail survey with a relatively large population of visually impaired individuals. Of course, the major caveat with the study cited here is that the population in question included a wide range of severity in terms of visual impairment. It is not clear whether such an approach would work with a population that is totally blind.

However, the implication of this study is that, in an era of constrained resources, less-expensive survey modes can indeed be used to conduct reliable and valid probability surveys with certain visually impaired populations.

Aknowledgements

The author wishes to thank the *New Jersey Commission for the Blind and Visually Impaired* for allowing these data to be used for public research and education and two anonymous reviewers for their helpful comments.

References

Braille Plus, Inc. nd. "Definition of Large Print." *Available at www.brailleplus.net*

Center for the Partially Sighted (CPS). nd. *Print Guidelines.* Available at *www.low-vision.org/large-print.html*

Craven, J. 2003. "Access to Electronic Resources by Visually Impaired People." *Information Research* 8(4), no. 156. Available at *informationr.net/ir/8-4/paper156.html*

Crudden, A. and McBroom, L.W. 1999. "Barriers to Employment: A Survey of Employed Persons Who are Visually Impaired." *Journal of Visual Impairment and Blindness*: June 1999 v.93:6.

Dillman, D.A. 1978. *Mail and Telephone Surveys: The Total Design Method.* New York: Wiley.

Eggett, C.B. 2002. "Assistive Technology Needs in Public Libraries: A Survey." *Journal of Visual Impairment and Blindness*: August 2002, pp.549-557.

Gerber, E. and Kirchner, C. 2001. "Who's Surfing? Internet Access and Computer Use by Visually Impaired Youths and Adults." *Journal of Visual Impairment and Blindness*: March 2001, pp.176-181.

Golledge, R.G. and Marston, J.R. 1997. "Attitudes of Visually Impaired Persons Toward the Use of Public Transportation." *Journal of Visual Impairment and Blindness*: Sept/Oct 1997, v.91:5.

Kitchel, J.E. 2001. "Large Print: Guidelines for Optimal Readability." American Printing House for the Blind. Available at *www.aph.org/edresearch/lpguide.htm*

Murray, P. 1997. *CBVI 1997 Voc Rehab Consumer Satisfaction Survey.* New Brunswick, NJ: Eagleton Institute Center for Public Interest Polling, Rutgers University.

Roundtable on Information Access. 2001. *Guidelines for the Production of Large Print (Summary)*. Melbourne, Australia.

Washington State Department of General Administration. nd. *Guidelines for Producing Materials in Large Print*. Available at *www.ga.wa.gov/ada/lgprint.htm*

In: Towards Best Practices for Surveying People..., Volume 1 ISBN 1-60021-195-X
Editors: Thilo Kroll, David Keer et al., pp. 181-215

Chapter 11

HOW TO REACH THE «INVISIBLE POPULATION» OF HARD OF HEARING AMERICANS

John G. Schroedel
University of Arkansas, Department of Rehabilitation, Human Resources, and Communication Disorders

ABSTRACT

That 22 million hard of hearing Americans comprise one of the most underresearched groups of persons with a disability underscores the need for this chapter. The first part of this chapter presents it's needs and objectives and defines the project's target population of persons with a hearing loss. The auditory and socio-demographic characteristics of these persons are described as are their employment patterns. Major flaws in prior research, such as a predominant prevalence of unrepresentative convenience samples, are identified. The attributes of social environments in which hard of hearing persons face difficulties in understanding speech are specified and proactive and reactive responsive coping styles are exemplified. Two theoretical research models were used for integrating diverse study variables. Patterns in knowing about and needing communication devices and workplace accommodations are elucidated. Variations in the severity of hearing loss were identified as a major influence upon many variables within the above listed topics. Examples of these variables are displayed in Figure 1.

The second part of this chapter depicts unique methods of project design and data collection. First, a nationwide sample of hard of hearing persons was identified via 66,000 random phone tracking calls. A follow-up mail survey yielded a first-ever comprehensive datafile on respondents' employment experiences and use of human services. Finally, the representativeness of the obtained mail sample was compared to results from a federal survey with benchmark attributes of the target population. The socio-demographic, geographic, auditory and other characteristics of the sample were compared to the characteristics of the population.

Key Employment Variables

<u>Worker Characteristics</u>

Education

Severity of Hearing Loss

Coping Styles

Occupation

<u>Characteristics of the Work Climate</u>

Supportive Boss

Supportive Co-workers

Need for Job Accommodations

<u>Outcomes</u>

Earnings

Job Satisfaction

Job Benefits

Figure 1.2

Stigmatizing Hearing Loss:

A Vicious Cycle and Self-Fulfilling Prophecy

"That's Stupid!"

Mishears

Underachieves

Misunderstands

Reduced Self-Esteem

Figure 1. Examples of variables

Needs for the Chapter

- Researchers need to better understand conditions such as why most hard of hearing persons prefer to be anonymous. This knowledge will enable social survey scientists to more readily identify these persons as prospective participants in studies and more accurately interpret the results from these studies.
- There is a crucial shortage of representative samples of hard of hearing persons. Most research studies on these individuals have used focus groups or interviewing from convenience samples. Because these research results cannot be generalized or inferred to other studies, the body of knowledge about the target population is fragmented. A convenience sample is a group of study participants readily accessible to the researcher, especially when other subjects are unavailable.
- Few research studies before 1990 focused on the psychological and vocational adjustment of hard of hearing adults. Schroedel (1984) analyzed 52 surveys of persons with hearing loss: 48 involved those deafened before age 19 and four involved those who were hard of hearing. Most research on adapting to mild to moderate hearing loss has been done in the previous 15 years, however, most studies are not readily accessible. Some research is available in consumer and professional journals, unfortunately, most documents are hard-to-retrieve research grant reports, conference presentations, and computerized on-line media.
- Almost no studies used theoretical models to organize research variables on hard of hearing persons so that more coherent findings can be developed. Furthermore, few studies have tested research hypotheses related to these individuals to yield more empirically valid and reliable research information.
- If more studies had included theoretical models and multivariate analyses, the subsequent knowledge base would be more integrated. However, few research studies have: (a) either identified the most important variables influencing findings or (b) explained why descriptive results have occurred. Lacking this decisive knowledge, researchers and research consumers can only make presumptions about the psycho-social and vocational adjustment of hard of hearing adults. This is a weak foundation for applying research results to improve services and set policies for these adults.
- Subsequently, hard of hearing Americans, the largest group of individuals with a chronic physical or sensory disability (Benson & Marano, 1994), are among the most under-researched groups of persons with a disability. The lack of empirical research on this population is especially notable considering it's demographic size. Why has this occurred? Communication or interaction mishaps due to a hearing loss can often be undetected, concealed, or avoided. Furthermore, few hard of hearing persons mingle together. These combined factors make these persons invisible on the radar screens of social scientists.

Objectives of the Chapter

- To identify the attitudes and behaviors of hard of hearing adults, such as denial of hearing loss, social withdrawal, and preferred anonymity, which bar participation of these individuals in social research studies.
- To report unprecedented research methods that led to obtaining the first-ever representative national sample of hard of hearing adults with in-depth information on their background characteristics and employment.
- To describe the significant contributions of project personnel and members of a national advisory panel, 70% of whom had a hearing loss, to the success of the project.
- So that social scientists can replicate this study key research procedures are fully reported and suggestions made for improving these procedures.
- Identify specific procedures to optimize inclusion of hard of hearing persons in future social research surveys.

This narrative reports on seven multi-step tasks which describe how the chapter Objectives were achieved.

Defining the Target Population

Twenty-one percent of the nation's population, or 54 million Americans, have a disability (U.S. Commission on Civil Rights, 1998). Among the estimated 29 million Americans with a hearing loss during 2004, 22.1 million were hard of hearing, 5.9 million deafened at or after age 19, and one million deafened before age 19 (Ries, 1994; Schroedel, Watson, & Ashmore, 2005; U.S. Census Bureau, 2003). This estimate is derived from the 1991 National Health Interview Survey (NHIS) which has the most reliable demographic data on hearing loss and used identical research methods in 1971, 1977, and 1991 (Ries, 1994). This 1971-1991 trend line in the number of Americans with hearing loss provides a benchmark to conservatively project these numbers to 2004 (Schroedel, Watson & Ashmore, 2005). Coincidentally, Kochkin (2001) independently determined that 28.6 million Americans had a hearing impairment in 2000.

In order to better understand hard of hearing individuals several groups with loss of hearing are defined. The 1991 NHIS describes a hard of hearing person as an individual who has a «reduced ability to usually hear and understand speech without a hearing aid» (Ries, 1994; Schein, 1996). By contrast, the NHIS defines a deaf person as one who «cannot hear and understand speech.» The issue if these definitions should include ability to hear with a hearing instrument is moot because only 20% of those needing hearing aids use them (Kochkin, 2001).

Recognizing the need to better define persons with hearing loss based upon functional limitations, the Rehabilitation Services Administration (RSA) in the U.S. Department of Education, developed a new disability coding system partially for the purpose of analyzing its nationwide case closure database (Reichman, 2001). George Kosovich (personal communication, January 20, 2005) and Tomlinson (1992) provided information to identify each code group below by more broadly understood terms. The following four codes represent most closed cases with a hearing impairment:

- *(03) Deafness: Communication Visual* in lay terms refers to deaf persons who use sign language.
- *(04) Deafness: Communication Auditory* comprises individuals with an unspecified age at onset and may commonly be identified as deaf persons who do not sign.
- *(05) Hearing Loss: Communication Visual* would generally be recognized as late-deafened persons or those who became deaf during adulthood. Because their hearing impairment began after the development of speech and language they can benefit from using English-based text technology such as communication access through real-time transliteration or computerized note taking. This group also has an unspecified age at onset of deafness.
- *(06) Hearing Loss: Communication Auditory* refers primarily to hard of hearing persons who use conventional modes of speech and hearing. These persons describe themselves with a hearing impairment ranging from mild to profound.

The RSA and NHIS definitions are related to the individual's capacity to comprehend spoken communication. Furthermore, the dependency on vision needed by many deaf persons compared to the dependency on auditory means by most hard of hearing persons is associated with many social and psychological differences between members of these two groups.

REVIEW OF THE LITERATURE

The literature review utilized three goals to facilitate achieving the objectives of this chapter. One goal is to identify gaps in what is known about essential variables which may yield useful information about hard of hearing persons. The second goal is to discover unknown variables which merit being added to the study. The third goal is to update knowledge on all relevant variables to more accurately understand and integrate them. The overall objective is to organize this information into a methodological design to obtain a representative sample of hard of hearing adults.

INDIVIDUAL CHARACTERISTICS

Auditory Characteristics:

Sampling significantly impacts upon information about the attributes of hearing loss among participants in various studies. More than two-thirds of the members of Self Help for Hard of Hearing People (SHHH) reported a severe to profound loss of hearing (Orlans & Meadow-Orlans, 1984; Sorkin, 1995). By contrast, three national studies of hearing-impaired persons determined that most had either a slight or mild loss (Kochkin, 1997; Ries, 1994; Schroedel, Watson, & Boone, 2004, May). These researchers used the Hearing Ability Scale, a Guttman response-scaled instrument with replies validated by audiometric records (see Methods section).

Other studies divulged that most afflicted persons started to lose their hearing during their prime working (35-64) years (Kyle & Wood, 1983; Orlans & Meadow-Orlans, 1984; Schroedel & Geyer, 1998). However, until recently there were no reliable surveys with nationwide representative samples, such as the National Health Interview Surveys, that provided accurate information on the age at onset among hard of hearing persons. Schroedel, Watson, and Boone (2004,May) were the first to report this information.

The literature on samples of adults who are hard of hearing or with adult-onset hearing loss is characterized by an almost total absence of objective criteria to evaluate severity of hearing impairment. Most hard of hearing persons have had neither a hearing test nor use hearing instruments (Kochkin, 2001). Objective criterion-referenced scales of the severity of hearing loss are seldom used. The most frequently utilized measures are either self-reported severity of hearing loss or self-identity as a person with a hearing loss. These conditions point to the need for cautious interpretation of research results across studies.

Socio-Demographic Characteristics

Various sources reveal important differences in this type of information. Studies show that members of national organizations of hard of hearing persons differ from their peers who do not join such groups. For example, members of SHHH were conspicuously older, better educated, less likely to be employed, and almost exclusively White (Sorkin, 1995) compared to broader samples of hard of hearing adults who are not members of organized consumer groups (Boone, Schroedel, Watson, & Anderson, 1996; El-Khiami, 1986; Market Opinion Research, 1989; Moore & Schroedel, 2000; Schroedel, Watson, & Boone, 2004,May).

It is vital to know important distinctions between various types of hard of hearing persons. A research team conducted a 15-year follow-up survey of alumni from colleges with comprehensive specialized service programs *for students with hearing loss* not usually found at regular institutions of higher education (El-Khiami, 1992, June; El-Khiami, 1993; Schroedel & Geyer, 1998, 2000). The team found that deaf college graduates consistently had higher educational and occupational attainments than their hard of hearing peers. However, it is crucial to recognize that the hard of hearing graduates in the long-term study differed from hard of hearing students from regular colleges, most of whom did not seek on-campus support services (Schroedel, Kelley, & Conway, 2002, 2003). Moreover, disproportionately more hard of hearing alumni in the 15-year study earned degrees from postsecondary vocational or technical training institutes, whereas their deaf counterparts more likely graduated from two-year and four-year academic programs (El-Khiami, 1992, 1993). Type of college significantly impacts the socioeconomic attainments of alumni with hearing loss (Schroedel, 1987; Schroedel & Watson, 1991).

Employment Patterns

Once again sampling confounds the generalizability of study findings. National surveys have documented confusing results on employment patterns among Americans with hearing loss. This problem, originating from surveys done by reputable social scientists, exemplifies the difficulties of research on this target population. Two standard statistics are involved:

- The *labor force participation rate.* Among those of working age (18-64) the labor force comprises workers and unemployed job seekers. Those not in the labor force include: retirees, homemakers, students, those too ill to work, or those who do not want to work.
- The *employment rate* is the percentage of those in the work force who have a job.

Ries (1994) calculated a 1991 labor force participation rate of 70% and an employment rate of 66% for adults with hearing loss more than 17 years of age. These rates essentially followed U. S. Bureau of the Census (1999) definitions. By contrast, another study reported that during 1983 58% of hearing-impaired adults participated in the labor force compared to 82% in 1993 and 59% in 1994 (Trupin, Sebesta, Yelin, & LaPlante, 1997). Parallel to this, an additional study determined that employment rates for workers with hearing loss were 64% in 1991-92, 65% in 1993-94, 64% in 1994-1995, and 62% in 1997 (Mc Neil, 2000). Note that in the former report the 1994 labor force participation rate (59%) was *lower* than the 1993-94 employment rate (64%) in the latter report, which excluded the probable 6% to 7% who were hearing-impaired unemployed job seekers.

Why did this happen? Both studies excluded persons more than 64 years of age, which contradicts Census Bureau definitions. This dilemma is problematic due to the increased prevalence of hearing loss as persons become older. In 1991 43% of all Americans with a hearing loss were more than 64 years of age, including about 12% of hearing-impaired workers (Ries, 1994). Also, differences in definitions of hearing loss, data collection procedures, and yearly sample sizes contributed to inconsistencies found in these reports other than Ries (1994). These conditions reinforce the need for more reliable research on the labor force participation, employment, and unemployment among these workers.

Characteristics of Communication Environments

Work, family, and other environments are filled with many pitfalls for hard of hearing persons. Particularly difficult situations for understanding spoken conversations among those with a mild or moderate hearing loss include: (a) participating in groups; (b) settings that are open, public, or noisy; (c) when the hearing-impaired listener is in an ineffectual physical listening position, involved with strangers, or with people in a hurry; and (d) using the telephone (Jaworski & Stephens, 1998; Kyle & Wood, 1985; Thomas, Lamont, & Harris, 1982).

Coping Behaviors

Many individuals who are hard of hearing or with an adult-onset hearing impairment face misunderstandings, interaction strain, and negative attitudes from hearing peers which lead to stress, reduced competency, diminished self-esteem, uncertainty, anxieties, communication fatigue, and depression (Hetu & Getty, 1993; Kerr & Cowrie, 1997; Kyle & Wood, 1985;

Meadow-Orlans & Orlans, 1990; Stika, 1997). These persons use either proactive or reactive coping styles to adjust to these adverse conditions (Hetu, 1993; Jaworski & Stephens, 1998; Knapp, 1948; Meadow-Orlans & Orlans, 1990; Schroedel, Kelley, & Conway, 2002, 2003; Stika, 1997). *Proactive styles* include: (a) assertiveness, (b)endeavoring harder than peers who hear, (c) speech reading, (d) asking for repetition, and (e) revealing the hearing loss. *Reactive styles* include: (a) denial, (b) pretense, (c) bluffing, (d) deception, (e) limited interaction, (f) faking understanding, (g) social withdrawal, (h) dominating a conversation so others cannot talk, and (i) using silence to prevent communication. Many of these reactive behaviors reflect resisting self-acceptance to being hard of hearing (Carmen, 2001). *There is no empirical evidence indicating that any specific set of these behaviors predominate among hard of hearing persons.*

Taken as a whole, these studies, although including many based upon convenience samples, explicitly show barriers to successful psychological and vocational adjustment. Furthermore, much less is known about the effective behavioral and communication strategies used by more typical hard of hearing adults, especially those who are younger in age (e.g., 18-44), of color, without a college education, and not members of special consumer organizations.

Theoretical Models of Coping in Diverse Environments

Two theories focus on specific factors which contribute to the adaptation by hard of hearing persons to various social and communication settings. One research model concentrates on the affects of stigmatizing attitudes by persons who hear which limit the achievements of hard of hearing individuals. The other research model centers on how those with acquired hearing loss manage spoken communication in order to effectively communicate in different situations.

A Social Psychological Model

This paradigm describes a *vicious cycle of stigma and a self-fulfilling prophecy* as diagramed in Figure 2. Viewing this figure from right to left, the essential actions in this model by hard of hearing individuals include: (a) mishearing then misunderstanding speech which lead to (b) reduced self-esteem, (c) social withdrawal, and (d) underachievement. Key reactions by some persons who hear include: (a) ridiculing a hard of hearing person in a socially awkward situation and (b) negatively viewing their underachievement which serves as a self-fulfilling prophecy of devaluating attitudes toward hard of hearing persons (Schroedel & Jacobsen, 1978; Stone & Colella, 1996). A pivotal concept in this theoretical model is a stigmatized stereotype which is a negative attitude based upon inexperience with the object of the attitude (Schroedel & Jacobsen, 1978). An instrumental factor in changing stigmatized stereotypes can be traced from the quality of the experiences, for example, hearing persons have with hard of hearing persons (Schroedel & Jacobsen, 1978; Stone & Colella, 1996). *Some* persons who are hard of hearing as well as *some* hearing counterparts often stigmatize loss of hearing. Many hard of hearing individuals deny or minimize the communicative and social disadvantages related to reduced ability to hear (Chartrand, 2000;

Hetu, Riverin, Getty, Lalande, & St. Cyr, 1990; Kyle, Jones, & Wood, 1985; Sorkin, 1997; Stika, 1997). This denial is expressed by avoidance, pretense, and other deceptive behaviors that mask anger, depression, and frustration. *It is essential to point out that not all persons who hear have negative attitudes or reactions toward hard of hearing individuals.*

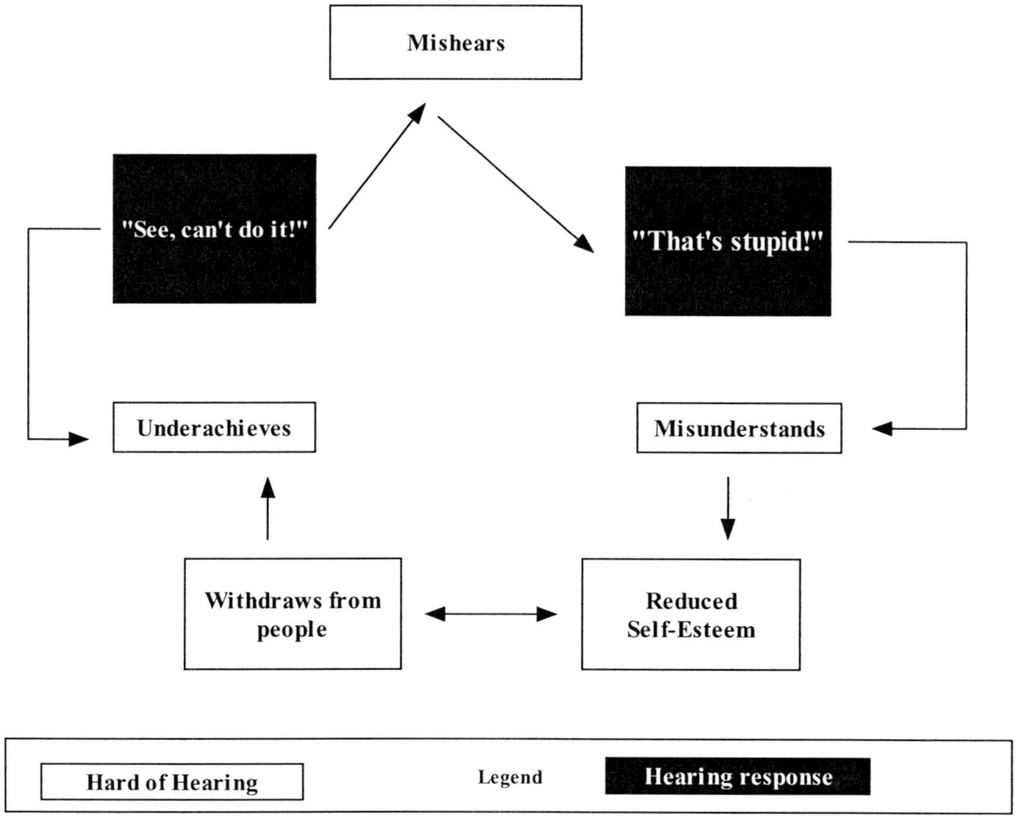

Figure 2. Stigmatizing Hearing Loss: A Vicious Cycle and Self-Fulfilling Prophecy.

A stigmatizing stereotype is more than an attitude held by an individual, rather, it is embedded in cultural values as a socially shared negative evaluation of people who are «different» (Balsamo, In press; Goffman, 1963). These stereotypes form a social psychological «master status» that often overrides the abilities of persons with disabilities (Schroedel & Jacobsen, 1978; Stone & Colella, 1996). In other words, these deeply rooted damaging stereotypes are difficult to change. To cope with these adverse attitudes most hard of hearing persons want to be seen as «normal» individuals without a disability. Relevantly, the prevalence of hearing loss increases as persons become older (Ries, 1994). Unfortunately, as the severity of the hearing loss worsens with passage of time, it becomes increasingly stressful to continue to act as a «person who can hear.» For example, how can such persons remain anonymous after frequently asking speakers to repeat what they said? Moreover, some stress related to deteriorating hearing ability can be self-inflicted. Balsamo noted that some persons who hear fuse stereotypes about hard of hearing people with stereotypes about deaf people. This contributes to the avoidance of many hard of hearing persons from attributes of deafness or deaf people such as sign language or specialized service programs for deaf persons (Schroedel, Kelley, & Conway, 2002, 2003).

Furthermore, depending upon the age at onset of their hearing loss, a hard of hearing persons may experience a lifetime of stigmatized stereotyping. Adolescents who disclosed their hearing loss were significantly more likely to be teased and bullied by hearing peers compared to students who did not reveal their hearing loss (Kent, 2003). Rigorous experiments with college students who hear found negative reactions toward attributes of impaired hearing such as behind-the-ear hearing aids and unintelligible speech (Blood, 1997; Casanova, Katkovsky, & Hershberger, 1988). Moreover, hearing workers tease and ridicule hearing-impaired workers (Hetu & Getty, 1993). These negative attitudes and behaviors by some hearing persons reinforce the denial adopted by many persons who are hard of hearing (Kochkin, 1993).

Dealing With Spoken Communication

Another research model addresses the question: how do persons who hear react to «invisible» adults with a mild hearing loss who consistently attempt to behave «normally» as nondisabled persons? The hearing loss exists as do consequent interaction and communication difficulties. Under these circumstances hard of hearing individuals attempt to *manage spoken information* (Kyle, Jones, & Wood, 1985). Essential components of spoken communication include: the rapidity, emotional intensity, and mental complexity of what is said. Because hearing loss reduces the ability to understand speech, the disadvantaged person must: (a) increase the level of control, (b) accept a reduced level of understanding, or (c) avoid situations where understanding is threatened. Many persons with a mild hearing loss, especially those without hearing instruments, experience situations which expose difficulties in communication and interaction. As expected, attributes of both the hearing-impaired person and the environment influence the level of adjustment. Kyle and Wood (1983) found that three-fourths of the individuals with a moderate adult-onset hearing impairment were uncomfortable in group conversations, public settings, and noisy surroundings. Diverse means were needed to reduce this discomfort and regain control of spoken communication (Kyle, Jones, & Woods, 1985).

Communication Devices and Environmental Accommodations

Knowing and using communication devices and related accommodations reduces disadvantages associated with hearing loss. Workers with moderate to profound hearing impairments reported home or work situations of communication deprivation, job limitations, manipulations by persons who hear, and distressed feelings (Kerr & Cowie, 1997). Another study of workers with acquired hearing loss stated they were generally satisfied with their jobs, but anxious about the effects of their hearing impairment upon future employment prospects (Kyle & Wood, 1985). They considered promotions to be curtailed and were content to work in anxiety-free unstimulating jobs with lower potential. Clearly, both individuals with and without hearing impairments contributed to these research results.

Modern technology evidently is not reaching many hard of hearing persons. Between 50% and 75% of members in a consumer group had assistive devices or workplace accommodations (Scherich, 1996; Sorkin, 1995). In a non-random study of hard of hearing adults about 40% owned special devices such as television captioning decoders and tele-text (TTD) phone devices (Harkins & Jensema, 1988). However, the representativeness of these samples is questionable. In contrast, a Michigan study, with a broader sample of hard of hearing persons, found that less than 25% used special devices (Market Opinion Research, 1989). During the past two decades among national samples of Americans with hearing loss only about 20% wore a hearing aid (Kochkin, 2001; Ries,1994; Weinstein, 1996). It could be surmised that the disinterest of most hard of hearing persons toward hearing instruments mirrors their disfavor of workplace accommodations. The research model on stigma implies that use of *visible* hearing aids or accommodations signal that the hard of hearing person is no longer either invisible or «normal.»

Most hard of hearing workers in one sample reported difficulties in work-related social functions, group meetings, in-service training, and socializing with co-workers (Scherich, 1996). Although a majority used assistive devices at work, few used support personnel (e.g., to answer the telephone) or changed their work duties (job restructuring). In other studies, many hard of hearing persons did not ask for on-the-job accommodations or use special equipment because they either feared unfavorable reactions from persons who hear or reacted negatively toward these devices (Bowe, 1991; Sorkin, 1997; Stika, 1997).

Severity of hearing loss is a pivotal factor in using on-the-job accommodations. Trybus, Stika, and Goulder (2004) reported on a national study of 400 workers, most of whom were severely hearing impaired. Except for a slight majority who used amplified phones or e-mail, less than 9% used any assistive technological devices. These researchers ascertained that the primary barriers to accepting and using on-the-job accommodations were *psychological concerns* such as fears of being singled out, stigmatized, or viewed as «different» from their hearing co-workers. A secondary factor was that 41% of participants were generally unfamiliar with these workplace accommodations. *The project data indicated that psychological barriers surmounted lack of knowledge about desiring and applying accommodations.* By contrast, in a nationally representative sample of hard of hearing workers less than 50% were aware of 16 of 19 on-the-job accommodations (Schroedel, Watson, & Boone, 2004, May). The only plausible explanation for these results is that: (a) some technological devices, such a computerized note taking, were unknown to most of these middle-aged workers or (b) wage earners in specific occupations did not need some accommodations and thus had no reason to know about them.

SUMMARY

This research review indicates that severity of the hearing loss is a crucial factor influencing communication and social interaction in various social settings. This creates a dilemma for researchers because many hard of hearing persons have a mild loss, but, most research studies used convenience samples primarily comprising adults with severe to profound impaired hearing. Subsequently, key characteristics of participants in various projects were carefully described throughout this review of the literature to set the extent to which research results may be generalized to other studies.

The literature, principally research on stigmatizing attributes of hearing loss, implies that adverse conditions prevail in the work place. However, two limitations accompany this statement. First, even though these attitudes exist, they do not spontaneously ignite negative behaviors toward persons with hearing loss. Second, the prevalence of these stigmatizing attitudes and behaviors representing unfair treatment is not known.

The research model of managing spoken communication was presented as an alternative approach to assess coping by mainly adults with a mild hearing loss in various social interactions. There are too many pitfalls in these social interactions for these persons to remain inconspicious and at some point their hearing associates will detect communication problems.

Various coping strategies comprise responses to conditions within interactive settings in order to communicate and act effectively. However, there is a scarcity of knowledge about how various coping techniques favorably change these settings. Research scientists and research consumers can implement this information to modify the attitudes and behaviors of hard of hearing adults to enhance their social integration and participation in research projects.

Hard of hearing persons comprise a sizable and heterogeneous group and mis-characterizing and stereotyping them must be avoided. Some hard of hearing persons act in certain ways, whereas others do not. Some factors such as using hearing aids, type of education, the severity of the hearing loss, and differences in the reactions of peers who hear were identified as key variables influencing the diverse attitudes and behaviors of hard of hearing persons.

The review of the literature accomplished its mission in compiling crucial information needed to overcome barriers which hinder the participation of hard of hearing adults in social surveys. Insights have been gained to help design research procedures to enhance prospects of obtaining a representative national sample of these persons. The state of knowledge is ripe to advance beyond convenience studies of this target population.

RESEARCH METHODS

The pioneering research methods used in this project have rarely, if ever, been previously employed in a study of Americans with hearing loss. To obtain a representative sample of an «invisible» population of hard of hearing adults required careful planning then implementing unique procedures to first locate then survey these persons. These procedures are described in sufficient detail to give the reader a clear understanding of how this was done.

This section outlines consecutive activities to plan, execute, and complete the project. First, a nationwide phone screening campaign was conducted to find a representative sample of 1,000 adults with hearing loss. Second, project staff verified the names and addresses obtained by the phone contacts to enhance the success of a follow-up mail survey. The third task was to design two respondent-friendly questionnaires for the survey to the 1,000 cases. Fourth, the survey data were reviewed, computer scanned, merged into databases, then analyzed.

The mail survey sample was evaluated to ascertain the extent to which it represented the nation's population of hard of hearing adults. Other national surveys were assessed to determine comparability across studies on the socio-demographic, geographic, and auditory attributes of survey participants. Obtaining a representative sample is essential for generalizing project results to other groups of hard of hearing adults. The chapter concludes with: (a) suggestions for enhancing participation of hard of hearing persons in social surveys, (b) recommendations for improving replication of this project's research procedures for future surveys, and (c) a chapter summary.

Objective 1. Identify a Representative National Sample of Hard of Hearing Adults

To guide project planning it was anticipated that 77% of the project sample would be hard of hearing, 20% deafened after age 19, and 3% deafened before age 19 (Ries, 1994). This information was obtained from the 1990-91 National Health Interview Survey (NHIS) which is the best available source of demographic information on hearing loss.

Task 1.1: Justifying National Telephone Screening

The telephone screening campaign followed a model (Taylor, Kagay, & Leichenko, 1986) used by Louis Harris and Associates in numerous major national telephone interviewing surveys of Americans with disabilities (e.g., Genevie, 1988; Kagay, 1987; Leitman, Cooner, & Risher, 1994; National Organization on Disability, 2000; Risher & Amorosi, 1998; Taylor, Kagay, & Leichenko, 1987; Taylor & Wurf, 1991). This approach enhanced the feasibility of acquiring a representative sample of the target population and removed the bias inherent in prior studies that have relied on mailing lists, focus groups, or interviewing members of consumer organizations.

Effectiveness

How effective is phone screening with persons with hearing loss? Two national surveys of hearing-impaired Americans determined that most had either a slight or mild hearing loss (Kochkin, 1997; Ries, 1994). National surveys also indicated that at least 95% of persons with and without hearing loss had telephones in 2001 (Ries, 1994; U.S. Bureau of the Census, 2003).

Relevantly, among Americans with a hearing loss the 3% who became deaf before age 19 are most likely than hard of hearing persons to have teletext phones or TDDs (Market Opinion Research, 1989; Miller Research Group, 1996; Ries, 1994). A review of TDD directories supported this conclusion (e.g., Arkansas Association of the Deaf, 2000; TDI, 2001). Two state studies successfully used computer-assisted random-dialed phone tracking of persons identified *10.1%* with a hearing loss (Market Opinion Research, 1989; Miller Research Group, 1996). These state prevalence rates were almost identical to the national prevalence rate of *9.7%* estimated in Schroedel, Watson, and Ashmore (2005). Taken as a whole, these research studies indicate that a large majority of persons in the target population use the telephone. *More important, phone screening is better than any other method, except for the very expensive National Health Interview Surveys, in producing a representative national sample of adults with hearing loss.*

Task. 1.2: Designing The Telephone Screening

The University of Arkansas Survey Research Center (SRC) in Fayetteville conducted the telephone screening. This nationwide activity consisted of two primary tasks:

First, SRC personnel designed a national survey sample representative of the nation's population of residential telephone users stratified by geographic region and metropolitan/non-metropolitan residence. Primary sampling units within this sampling frame were then selected through multistage unclustered sampling of states then smaller geographic divisions.

Second, household phone numbers in primary sampling units were generated through random dialing procedures. The main purpose of the phone screening was to identify the hearing status of persons called through questions listed in the Phone Screening Script (See enclosure at end of chapter).

Task 1.3: Determining the Number of Phone Calls Needed

Several salient criteria were used to determine the scope of work for the telephone screening:

Demographic criterion: We conservatively estimated that *an average 9%* (range: 8.3% to 9.1%) of the American population had a hearing loss in 2000 (National Center for Health Statistics, 1998; Ries, 1985, 1994; Schein, 1996). Thus, calls to 11 households will yield one person with a hearing impairment. This prevalence rate was an underestimate as «insurance» to assist in obtaining the targeted 1,000 persons.

Telephone Refusal Rate: An accurate estimate was needed of those who would refuse to cooperate with the phone screener. Dated phone interviewing studies reported that between 17% and 21% of persons with disabilities refused to be interviewed (Kagay, 1987; Taylor, et al., 1986). However, proliferation of telemarketing and caller ID devices clearly indicates that a much higher refusal rate was required (See below).

Mail Survey Refusal Rate: We estimated that approximately 30% of persons with hearing loss would decline to participate in the follow-up mail survey. This 30% is above the midpoint between 17% and 38% of prospective respondents who refused to cooperate with follow-up mail surveys in two state phone screening studies (Market Opinion Research, 1989; Miller Research Group, 1996). The 17% refusal rate from a phone study conducted in Oklahoma suggests that the 30% refusal rate may be an overestimate (Boone, Schroedel, Watson, & Anderson, 1996).

Call Backs: Up to three call backs were made to numbers initially busy or not answered. One call back was made to persons who «softly» refused a previous call.

Task 1.4: Specifying the Numbers of Phone Calls Needed

The project team collaborated with SRC personnel to calculate that 66,400 phone calls would be needed to canvas households in order to identify the 1,000 adults for the sample:

- An initial 11,100 calls would be required to reach the targeted 1,000 persons.
- Based upon actual phone interviewing experience SRC managers computed that 50% of these 11,100 calls would be refused, requiring an additional 11,100 calls (for a total of 22,200 calls) to find 1,000 Americans with hearing loss willing to complete the phone tracking questions.
- To compensate for the 30% declining to participate in the follow-up mail survey, an extra 9,500 calls would be required. This raised the total number of calls to 31,700.

- An estimated 20% of these 31,700 calls would be busy answers, no answers, or answering machines. This added another 7,900 calls to overcome this factor for a total of 39,700 calls.
- An estimated 52% of the telephone calls would be to non-operative numbers, necessitating another 43,300 calls for a total of 83,000 numbers. Non-operative numbers included disconnects, fax machines, computer/LSD lines, pagers, cell phones, and business (nonresidential) phones. The master tape of 103,000 phone numbers was not expected to have any business lines, however, the owners of phone numbers do change rapidly after being disconnected, thus a former home number can become a business number.
- An estimated 80% of these 83,000 numbers would be reached, meaning an actual total of 66,400 calls was dialed.

Task 1.5: Preparing Screening Operations

- **Phone Tracking Script:** A 11-question script for the telephone tracking was extensively pilot tested, revised, then approved by the University's Institutional Review Board to ensure compliance with informed consent procedures (see attachment at end of chapter).
- **Training Supervisors:** Project personnel trained the supervisors of the SRC phone trackers so that the latter would be conversant with the phone screening script. Also screeners were instructed to decrease potential participant resistance by: (a) clearly explaining the purposes of the research study, (b) stressing the importance of informed consent, and (c) emphasizing the confidentiality of the project data.
- **TDD and Fax Calls:** The screeners were also trained to detect the difference between a TDD and a fax machine, a difficult task for an inexperienced person. The SRC sent a list of more than 100 «possible» TDD numbers to the project team who decided it would be counter productive to test them. Only a very experienced 711 relay phone operator can distinguish between fax and TDD calls. The few cases expected to be TDDs would be for deaf persons, not hard of hearing persons. In short, the time required to verify these phone numbers would have been counterproductive. The chapter author has found TDD follow-ups in prior mail surveys to very time consuming and generating few completed mailed survey forms (e.g., Geyer & Schroedel, 1999a, 1999b; Schroedel & Geyer, 2000; 2001).
- **Enhancing Representativeness of the Sample:** Procedures were made to ensure equal participation, especially for African-Americans and Latinos. Spanish-speaking phone trackers were employed on all work shifts. In addition, because the focus of this research project was upon employment of persons with hearing loss, steps were taken to maximize identifying workers. As allowed by the sampling design, calling on Monday through Thursday evenings and weekends when workers were more likely to be at home was emphasized.

- **RT-31 Monitoring of Screening:** Each week the SRC prepared a progress report on completed activities and encouraged the project team to visit the Center to review these activities and confer with the tracking managers.

Task 1.6: Phone Screening Conducted

From October 26 to November 21, 2001 and from January 1 to March 30,2002, except for a planned holiday pause, 121 trackers placed 66,400 calls to identify 1,050 adults who met the sampling criteria and *exceeded the planned target of 1,000 cases.* This schedule was the best window of opportunity to achieve the highest «hit rate» of prospectively eligible persons when they would be much more likely to be at home and, in turn, maximize the cost effectiveness of the phone screening.

Several notable patterns emerged during the phone screening:

- **Trouble Shooting:** With an average «hit rate» of one identified person with hearing loss for approximately every 63 calls, careful efforts were made to uphold the morale of the phone trackers during this tedious task. For example, project personnel visited the Survey Research Center and weekly congratulated the most productive phone trackers identified by SRC supervisors.
- **Miscommunications While Phoning:** Errors can occur during telephone conversations between persons who hear and persons with a hearing loss. The only data available to exemplify this problem was derived from a 3-week period in which phone trackers recorded that 127 hearing-impaired persons declined to participate because they misunderstood the purpose of the survey, felt they were too old, or did not want to receive mail during the anthrax postage scare. Other distrusted the approach of the phone tracking as a «pitch» to telemarket hearing aids. Probably others perceived that a survey from the University of Arkansas was totally irrelevant to them. The increased estimate of the percentage of persons refusing phone calls compensated for these problems.

Task 2: Preparing for the Mail Survey

Getting ready for the national mail survey required two major activities: (a) corroborating the names and addresses on the SRC list and (b) preparing consumer-friendly survey questionnaires.

- **Verifying the Mailing List:** It is known that an inaccurate or obsolete mailing list can reduce a survey response rate by more than 22% and inflate the sampling margin of error (Schroedel, 1984). Reports of miscommunications during the phone screening phase convinced the project team to verify the names and addresses on the SRC list. Mail may achieve what phone calling could not as 97%t of those with acquired hearing loss read daily compared to 60% of persons who hear (Kyle, Jones, & Wood, 1985). Three waves of contact letters were mailed to the 1,050 persons on this list. These letters included a mail-back form asking persons to: (a) make needed changes in their names or addresses, (b) update their work status, and (c) indicate if they needed a large print questionnaire. Another purpose of these letters was to make the project more familiar to prospective survey respondents to induce their cooperation. Among those who replied to the letters 52 requested large-print survey forms. Due to the increased prevalence of hearing loss and vision loss as persons get older these large-print questionnaires were needed.
- **Reasons for Deactivating Some Cases:** These mailings created many initially undelivered letters that had to be resolved by reverse phone tracking and Zip

book checking of names and addresses. The success of this process was enhanced by updating files on all problem cases to document information for project staff decisions to include or exclude persons on the master list. Actions for tracking prospective survey respondents and verifying their names and addresses followed standard practices (Call, Otto, & Spenner, 1982; Clarridge, Sheehy, & Hauser, 1976; King & Thorne, 1977). As a result of these and related activities 192 persons (18%) were deactivated from the SRC list of 1,050 cases. These deletions included:

- 96 cases with uncorrectable names and/or addresses despite maximum efforts to make them potential respondents.
- 47 cases in which it was not clear who in the household had a hearing loss (the key person). These situations probably stemmed from confusion due to either proxy- assisted calls or the proxy respondent not informing the key person about the screening call. Without a correct person's name, follow-up letters were not feasible. It was decided that because additional phone calls would not find a sufficient number of correctly identified key persons, these cases were deleted.
- 37 persons were classified as ineligible for the mail survey due to self-reported or proxy reported conditions such as they were: (a) institutionalized, (b) too ill to cooperate, (c) had no hearing loss, (d) deceased, or (e) victims of pranks.
- 12 persons lacked information on their current employment status because they had not responded to the contact letters. Because there were two survey questionnaires, one for those employed and another for those not now employed, these cases were deactivated.
- Consequently, 858 persons remained on the updated mailing list. These included 91.5% self-identified as hard of hearing and 8.5% self-identified as deaf, proportions similar to those found in the Oklahoma telephone screening survey (Boone, et al., 1996).
- One other advantage of the verification process is that without these mailings almost 100 unidentified problem cases would have remained on the SRC mailing list and subsequently reduced the response rate to the mail survey. Information on most of the 192 excluded cases came from either responses to the contact letters or undeliverable letters for which correct addresses could be not located.

Task 3: Data Collection Activities Planned and Completed

Three key activities were necessary to plan and accomplish this task: (a) design two questionnaires, (b) convene meetings of a national panel of expert specialists, and (c) conduct the mail survey.

Task 3.1: Questionnaires Prepared

Two 12-page mail survey forms, one for those working and the other for those not now working, were prepared by the project team. Two questionnaires were needed because some different items were aimed at each target group and separate questionnaires would be less lengthy and easier for survey participants to follow. Survey forms from ten prior studies of convenience samples of hard of hearing adults were reviewed to identify appropriate questions. The survey forms were peer reviewed by: (a) RT-31 research faculty, (b) the Prime Study Group, and (c) SRC personnel. After the survey forms were pilot tested with hard of hearing adults, the revised questionnaires were approved by the University's Institutional Review Board for meeting compliance with informed consent procedures. The project team and SRC staff formatted two scannable 12-page survey forms and SRC personnel prepared corresponding code books.

Task 3.2: Convene Meetings of the Prime Study Group (PSG)

To enhance the relevancy and quality of the project eight nationally recognized experts on the vocational rehabilitation and employment of hard of hearing persons met with Center research faculty and SRC staff on March 6-7, 2002 and October 21-23, 2003. Seventy percent of attendees had a hearing loss and contributed both personal insights and professional expertise to the group. The panelists improved the survey questionnaires by selecting items to match research priorities and suitability for respondents. They also clarified definitions of variables and presented ideas to make communicating research results more consumer friendly. Furthermore, PSG members identified key national issues in delivery of vocational rehabilitation services to hard of hearing consumers and actions needed to improve training of specialized counselors to serve this consumer group. These activities are among the main long-term outcomes of the overall project. This early cooperation between service professionals as research consumers and researchers enhanced the utility of the survey results.

Task 3.3: Data Collection Conducted

Between October 3 and November 15, 2002 three waves of the survey questionnaires were mailed out. Each mailing was accompanied by a carefully crafted covering letter to encourage responses to the survey. Returned survey forms were logged by respondent's ID number to control the mailings. The first mailing sent to 778 persons with verified addresses yielded 192 completed questionnaires for a 25.1% reply rate. Wave two, supplemented by other cases with corrected addresses, was mailed to 716 persons and 77 (11.3%) usable questionnaires came back. Wave three was sent to 597 cases and harvested 44 (7.8%) completed survey forms. Further mailings were ended because of diminishing response rates and the approaching holidays. The database comprised 313 usable questionnaires. The overall response rate to the mail survey was 36.5%.

Task 4: Review Returned Questionnaires and Setup Databases

These activities ensured that the survey database was error-free as feasible and organized to optimize data retrieval.

Task 4.1 Questionnaires Reviewed

The project team reviewed respondent's answers to each question in the 313 survey forms to correct unallowable or inaccurate replies, such as clarifying unreadable answers, violations of skip instructions, or what is known as a response set (e.g., circling one entire response column in a list of questions instead of replying to each item). Note that in many sets of questions positive items were alternated with negative items to induce diverse response patterns. Thus, response sets were clearly evident. All corrected errors were recorded to assist SRC staff scanning the questionnaires.

Task 4.2: Use of SRC Deliverables

The SRC then provided the project team with code books and frequencies for items in the two questionnaires. Other SRC deliverables included: (a) the final master list of names and addresses and (b) disk as well as hard copy frequencies of responses to all questions on the telephone screening script. Project personnel used these materials to organize databases to assess the representativeness of the obtained mail sample, the first and most important step in the analyses of the data.

Task 4.3: Databases Organized

To test the representativeness of the survey sample a multistage procedure united data from the «Your Job Now» survey form and the «Your Life Now» survey form. The first form was for 121 respondents currently employed during the survey. The second form included: (a) 90 persons whose employment ended at some point during the 1990s, and (b) 102 persons with no employment history after 1991 and thus retired. The two databases for the survey forms, each with a different sequence of questionnaire item numbers, were perfectly matched for 237 variables.

Task 4.4: The Hearing Ability Scale

This scale was a crucial tool in evaluating the representativeness of respondent's hearing loss in the project sample (see Table 5 below). The HAS was the most important measure used in this project because it provided the best reliable and valid assessment of the severity of hearing loss which was the most significant independent variable in the study. This scale contains four statements about the ability to hear: (a) a whisper, (b) a normal voice, (c) a shout, and (d) someone speaking loudly into your ear. Each person replies either Yes or No to each statement. The HAS, known as a Guttman scale, requires the respondent to make an orderly, thus scaled pattern of replies. Responding Yes to hearing a shout, but No to hearing a normal voice is not a scaled response. This measure has a 90% scaled response rate and correlates at .74 with audiometric measures of hearing loss (Schein, 1968; Schein, Gentile, & Haase, 1965). It has been used in the most reliable NHIS surveys on persons with hearing loss in the United States since 1971 (Ries, 1994). However, as we learned, it is best used in household interviewing where the trained interviewer can assist the interviewee to better understand the scale to avoid undercounting true cases of hearing loss. It was less effective in this mail survey as only 54% of the respondents (190 of 313) gave Guttman-scaled response patterns. However, it is much more objective than a four-item self-report measure of the severity of hearing loss modified from Orlans and Meadow-Orlans (1984).

Task 5: Assessing the Representativeness of the Sample

According to sampling theory, representativeness is determined by the extent to which the proportion of an attribute in the sample corresponds to the proportion of the same attribute in the population from which the sample was drawn. In a sample of 350-400 respondents a proportion of 50% will have a margin of sampling error of plus or minus 5.5% at the 95% level of confidence (Fowler, 1984). This means that there is a 95% probability that the comparable proportion in the population will be between 44.5% and 55.5%. Doubling the size of the sample to 800 respondents will only reduce the margin of error to 3.5%. Thus, a sample of about 350 cases will have an acceptable rate of sampling error acquired at a reasonable financial cost. The estimated margin of error for the 2002 mail survey sample was +/-5% for all 313 respondents.

SOCIODEMOGRAPHIC REPRESENTATIVENESS

The 1991 National Health Interview Survey (Ries, 1994) was the last and only federal survey that used *a series of instruments*, including the HAS, to assess hearing loss, making it the best demographic resource available. Therefore, characteristics of the project sample were compared with corresponding attributes from the 1991 NHIS population, as shown in Table 1. These comparisons were very similar for 5 of 8 synonymous characteristics assessed: age, gender, race, non-Hispanic origins, and martial status. Three disparities were due to differences in data collection methods mainly because the project sample was from a mail survey whereas NHIS data were from household interviewing. There was a higher percentage of white-collar workers in the 2002 sample, a condition known as upward socioeconomic response bias which can occur in mail surveys (Schroedel, 1984). Due to the telephone screening, the sample had a higher percentage of persons with a hearing loss after 19 years of age and a smaller proportion of those living with relatives, presumably hearing, who could help with phone calls. The 1991 NHIS had no comparable data on education. The 2002 telephone screening covered 48 states; Alaska and Hawaii were excluded due to high phone expenses. The phone screening obtained addresses from 48 states and the mail survey obtained questionnaires from 43 states.

Table 1. Comparing Selected Characteristics of Obtained 2002 Project Sample with 1991 National Health Interview Survey (NHIS)

Characteristics	2002 Sample	1991 NHIS*
Average age in years	62.3	62.0
Male	61.0%	61.4%
White	90.4%	90.2%
Non-Hispanic origins	91.0%	92.1%
Professional, managerial, and technical workers	36%	29%
Sales, clerical, and service workers	31%	31%
Trades workers, machine operators, laborers	33%	40%
Average completed education	some college	N/A**
Married	67.6%	66.7%
Live with relatives	65.0%	75.3%
Onset of hearing loss after age 19	87.7%	80.1%
Number of states contacted	43 of 48	50

*Source: Ries (1994)

**The 1991 NHIS reported three categories of obtained education: (a) less than 12 years, (b) 12 years, (c) more than 12 years. These gross categories were incomparable to the 8 degree-related categories of educational attainment used in the 2002 mail survey.

GEOGRAPHICAL REPRESENTATIVENESS

Table 2 illustrates the distributions of respondents in the four Census Bureau regions for the 2002 sample compared to samples in four NHIS surveys between 1991 and 2001. Participants in the 2002 sample survey and the 1996, 1998, and 2001 NHIS surveys were most evenly distributed in the Northeast and Midwest regions and a bit less equally spread across the South and West regions. Because of general population shifts across time, the outdated geographical distribution in the 1991 NHIS sample is less comparable to the 2002 sample.

Table 2. Percent Distribution of Hard of Hearing Persons by Region in Five National Surveys

Region	1991 NHIS	1996 NHIS	1998 NHIS	2001 NHIS	2002 Survey*
Northeast	16	18	16	17	19
Midwest	27	25	30	29	26
South	33	34	34	34	30
West	24	23	20	20	25
Total	**100**	**100**	**100**	**100**	**100**

Census Bureau regions: Northeast: ME, VT, NH, MA, CN, RI, NY, NJ, PA; Midwest: OH, IL, IN, MI, WI, MN, IO, MO, ND, SD, KS, NE; South: DE, MD, DC, WV, VA, KY, TN, NC, SC, GA, FL, AL, MS, LA, OK, AR, TX; West: WA, OR, CA, NV, AZ, ID, UT, CO, MT, WY, AK, HI.

Sources: Adams, Hendershot, & Marano (1999); Lucas, Schiller, & Benson (2004), Plies & Coles (2002); Ries, (1994) * N = 312 persons in 2002 national survey of hard of hearing adults

One condition impacted the proportions of residents with hearing loss in the four Census regions. This refers to the geographic density of these individuals, meaning the ratio of hearing-impaired Americans per 100,000 of the general population, which varies across regions and over time. For example, Schein and Delk (1974) reported that the 1971 density of persons with hearing loss was highest in the West (7,170 per 100,000) and lowest in the Northeast (5,977 per 100,000). Or, in other terms, about 72 per 1,000 in the West and 60 per 1,000 in the Northeast. However, due to differences in defining hearing loss in the NHIS surveys, except for 1971, 1977, and 1991, there was less reliable data to report changes in regional population densities after 1991 (see Table 2 below). For 1991 Ries determined that the smallest proportion of hearing-impaired persons resided in the Northeast compared to the largest proportion who lived in the South, after adjusting for the size of the general population in each region. These data imply a decline in the population with hearing loss in the Northeastern states between 1971 and 1991, which began in the 1960s (Schein & Delk, 1974).

Another method of assessing the representativeness of the 2002 mail survey sample is comparing geographical distribution of the respondents to the 1,050 persons on the SRC master address list resulting from *random* phone calls. This is displayed in Tables 3A and 3B. The geographical spread of mail survey respondents and those on the SRC telephone list are most similar in the West, Midwest, and Northeast regions. There were disproportionately fewer mail survey respondents living in the South compared to those on the SRC phone list, primarily due to fewer mail survey participants from Florida and Texas. Persons of Hispanic origins in these two states were not a factor in the under-representation of respondents (see Table 1) partially because Spanish-speaking phone trackers were on every work shift.

Table 3

Table 3A Comparing Contact Results: Percentages by States

State	Telephoning Results	Obtained Questionnaire Results
Washington	2.3%	3.5%
Oregon	1.0%	1.0%
California	10.8%	9.6%
Idaho	0.4%	0.0%
Nevada	0.3%	0.3%
Montana	0.6%	0.0%
Wyoming	0.3%	1.0%
Utah	1.5%	2.2%
Colorado	2.0%	2.6%
Arizona	2.2%	2.6%
New Mexico	0.8%	1.0%
West Regional Total	22.2%	23.8%
North Dakota	0.4%	0.0%
South Dakota	0.2%	0.3%
Nebraska	0.5%	1.0%
Kansas	1.0%	0.6%
Minnesota	1.7%	2.9%
Iowa	1.6%	2.6%
Missouri	3.3%	3.2%
Wisconsin	1.3%	1.9%
Illinois	3.9%	4.5%
Michigan	3.9%	3.5%
Indiana	2.3%	2.6%
Ohio	3.8%	3.5%
Mid-West Regional Total	23.9%	26.6%

Table 3B Comparing Contact Results: Percentages by States

State	Telephoning Results	Obtained Questionnaire Results
Maine	0.6%	1.3%
New Hampshire	0.9%	1.6%
Vermont	0.4%	0.0%
Massachusetts	1.8%	2.2%
Rhode Island	0.3%	0.3%
Connecticut	1.0%	1.6%
New York	5.1%	5.1%
Pennsylvania	4.5%	3.8%
New Jersey	2.2%	3.2%
Northeast Regional Total	16.8%	19.1%

Table 3: continued

Table 3B Comparing Contact Results: Percentages by States		
State	Telephoning Results	Obtained Questionnaire Results
Maryland	1.2%	0.3%
Virginia	1.5%	0.3%
West Virginia	0.9%	1.3%
Kentucky	1.5%	1.3%
North Carolina	2.4%	2.2%
South Carolina	2.0%	1.6%
Georgia	2.5%	2.6%
Florida	5.6%	2.9%
Tennessee	3.2%	2.2%
Alabama	2.3%	3.5%
Mississippi	1.4%	1.0%
Arkansas	2.3%	1.9%
Louisiana	0.9%	1.0%
Texas	7.0%	5.8%
Oklahoma	2.3%	2.6%
South Regional Total	37.0%	30.5%

Comparisons between the two lists in these tables present very similar proportions of participants within corresponding pairs of states. Completed mail questionnaires were received from 43 states and in 37 there was a difference of one percentage point or less between the corresponding proportions of persons contacted by phone and the mail survey. For example, New York had 5.1% of all persons contacted by phone and 5.1% of mail survey respondents. Likewise, Mississippi had 1.4% of those contacted by phone and 1.0% of those submitting questionnaires. Overall, these comparisons suggest that the completed mail sample was geographically comparable to the SRC master address list.

Auditory Representativeness

Survey participants were similar to those in other national studies regarding the severity of their hearing impairments. Because variation in severity of hearing loss is a crucial factor in communication and social interaction, a key question is: what is the range in hearing loss within this sample? *Self-reported information* is displayed in Table 4 based upon persons from two national surveys who did not use personal listening devices. It is known that only 22% of hearing-impaired Americans use hearing instruments (Kochkin, 2001). Both samples had fairly diverse distributions in the severity of their hearing loss except the project sample included a larger percentage of adults with severe and profound hearing loss. Other variations in these responses probably stemmed from differences in the ways these questions were asked.

Table 4. Percent Distribution of Self-Reported Severity of Hearing Loss With and Without Using a Personal Listening Device

Severity of Hearing Loss	2002 Sample*	1997 Sample**
Mild	26	72
Moderate	49	21
Severe	23	7
Profound	2	
Total	100	100

* N = 190 workers in project sample. ** Kochkin (1997) N = projected from 5,954 cases.

To achieve a more objective assessment of severity of hearing loss, responses to the Hearing Ability Scale (HAS) by persons in the project sample and the 1991 NHIS are presented in Table 5. The results in this table are congruent with those in Table 4: the 2002 survey group included disproportionately more persons with a severe hearing impairment than those in the 1991 NHIS. This information is derived from the 190 of 313 respondents in the 2002 sample who gave Guttman-scaled responses to the HAS (54%); 123 others did not give scalable replies. In addition, because a standard measure of hearing loss was utilized, the results across samples in Table 5 are more consistent than in Table 4. Moreover, there is no evidence of systematic bias, such as less education or increased age among survey participants, influencing erroneous replies to the HAS.

Table 5. Percent Distribution of Replies to the Hearing Ability Scale By Two Samples of Respondents

Hearing Situations	2002 Sample	1991 NHIS*
Can hear normal voice and whispers	61	69
Can hear shout	29	25
Can hear loud speech	2	3
Deaf	8	3
Total	100	100

* Ries (1994) N = estimated 20,600 interviewees

Note: Most items included hearing in "a quiet room" which is an optimal communication setting.

Some Americans have a bilateral loss of hearing in both ears, whereas others have a unilateral loss of hearing in one ear. As seen in Table 6, 71% of the mail survey respondents had a bilateral hearing impairment compared to 57% in the 1991 NHIS. Part of this discrepancy is due to increased prevalence of bilateral hearing loss since 1971 (Ries, 1994). However, the 2002 survey group had a larger percentage with a lot of trouble hearing in both ears than the corresponding 1991 NHIS group. The results in Table 6 coincide with those in Tables 4 and 5: the mail survey sample included disproportionately more severely hearing-impaired individuals than found in other samples. In Table 6 one-fourth of the workers had a unilateral hearing impairment in contrast to 37% in the 1991 NHIS. Four percent in each sample reported having «good hearing» yet participated in the study which indicated a borderline hearing loss. Both studies used the same self-report measure of ability to hear in each ear taken from the 1990-91 NHIS.

Table 6. Percent Distribution of Bilateral and Unilateral Hearing Loss In Two National Samples

Category of Hearing Loss	2002 Survey	1991 NHIS*
A lot of trouble hearing in both ears**	25	13
A little trouble hearing in both ears	46	44
Unilateral hearing loss	25	37
Good hearing in both ears**	4	4
Total	100	100

N = 197 hard of hearing workers.

* Source: Ries (1994)

** A few deaf respondents were combined with those with a lot of trouble hearing.

Task 6: Enhancing Inclusion of Hard of Hearing Persons In Surveys

Task 6.1: During the Phone Tracking

The phone tracking identified 1,050 American adults with hearing loss, which exceeded it's goal of 1,000 cases. Moreover, as shown in Tables 4-6, the mail survey sample included about 10% more severely to profoundly hearing-impaired persons than found in other national surveys. Thus, the phone tracking successfully included this group. Several crucial decisions augmented the effectiveness of the phone tracking:

- We learned that prior state phone-tracking studies competently located and identified expected proportions of hard of hearing and deaf adults. The question became: How could this be done at the national level?
- That question became: How many phone call would be needed to find 1.000 adults with hearing loss willing to participate in a follow-up mail survey? Key variables such as demographic prevalence rates as well as estimated rates for telephone refusals and mail survey refusals were added to a formula including estimates of non-operative phone numbers (e.g., faxes, voice boxes, pagers, and cell phones) and the number of reachable phone numbers(e.g., live household lines, telephone not busy, and «soft» refusals). It was computed that 66,400 calls were needed to reach 1,000 targeted cooperative cases.
- The telephone tracking script was extensively piloted tested during one-on-one interviews with local hard of hearing persons by project staff and in numerous telephone trials by SRC staff. This led to many improvements in the script.
- Spanish-speaking trackers worked during all shifts of the phone tracking.
- Hearing proxy respondents were allowed to answer questions for persons with difficulties understanding telephone calls. The advantages and disadvantages of this procedure were weighed toward facilitating their inclusion. Unexpectedly, some proxy respondents did not inform the household member with a hearing loss about the SRC phone call which confused that member after receiving survey mailings. A corrected note should be added to the next version of the phone script.
- Dispirited phone trackers can make errors which compound communication problems with some hearing-impaired phone listeners, which would discourage their

participation in the survey. Careful efforts were made to maintain the morale of these trackers by regular visits by leading project staff and weekly recognition of the most productive trackers.

Task 6.2: Conducting The Mail Survey

Many actions were taken to improve involving hard of hearing persons in the mail survey:

- Three mailings of initial contact letters and three mailings of survey questionnaires were conducted. Many mail surveys to deaf and hard of hearing adults do not attempt this many mailings (e.g., Schroedel, 1984).
- Because the prevalence of vision and hearing loss increase with getting older, the initial contact letters included a mailback sheet asking, among other questions, if the prospective respondent needed a large-print questionnaire; 52 persons said yes.
- An accurate mailing list enhances the final survey response rate resulting in a larger sample with a lower sampling margin of error. The various mailings revealed problem cases that were throughly and systematically checked. Updated records of such cases enabled project personnel to judiciously delete 192 cases, half with uncorrectable names and addresses, from the project's master mailing list. These steps also saved the time of project staff because the list verification status as eligible, ineligible, or pending of every person was current. Indecisive or delayed communication could convert a possible respondent to a definite refusal.
- The survey questionnaires were aptly crafted. Survey forms from 10 previous studies of hard of haring persons were examined to identify appropriate items. To encourage respondent participation, two 12-page survey forms were developed, one for those working now, and another for those not working now. One long questionnaire with many skip instructions between items would severely impair the survey response rate. The best available professionals, most of whom had a hearing loss, reviewed the questionnaires by «thinking hard of hearing» to improve the language, questions, and formatting of the questionnaires.
- Although only 36% replied to the mail survey, prudent comparisons to other national surveys, especially the 1990-1991 NHIS, concluded that the mail sample was representative of the nation's population of hard of hearing adults. Moreover, the number of respondents (N = 313) resulted in an acceptable margin of sampling error.

Task 7: Toward Better Replication from Lessons Learned

- Project personnel applied rigorous scientific research methods and sound professional judgment. However, at times this pioneering project ventured into uncharted territory with few guidelines to resolve uncertain issues in research design or methods. Consequently, several valuable lessons learned during the course of this project are worth recording so that future researchers can better replicate the study.
- A major improvement would have been to change the sequence of several major tasks in the project. One would have been to complete the survey questionnaires before starting the phone screening. A second would have the SRC provide the project team with 100 names and addresses at a time instead of waiting for the final list of 1,050 persons. Thus, mailings could have been done much sooner after the

SRC identified cooperative prospective respondents. An unknown number of probable respondents who would have completed questionnaires were lost due to the delay between phone and mail contacts. However, this piecemeal approach requires: (a) closely coordinating the multiple mailings of initial contact letters and survey questionnaires and (b) meticulous logging of results from these mailing waves. Prospective participants delayed responding for weeks while a next mailing was disseminated, thus late respondents would fall between the cracks without accurate and current records of their survey participation status

- Conducting these time-consuming tasks must consider a project's finite resources. One exemplary complication is while many prospective respondents delay for weeks before answering a survey mailing, the survey team must prepare a next mailing wave. This situation intensifies the need for accurate and timely records of the response status of targeted persons to various mailings. When a potential participant is classified as «reply pending,» project staff must enclose a special covering letter to all such cases stating, «in the event you have not answered us here is another copy for you to reply.» This method of precisely identifying subgroups of potential respondents for the next mailing wave solves several problems: (a) a targeted person's incoming reply crossing in the mail with the team's outgoing document will not aggravate this person if he or she gets an additional mailing and (b) persons who set aside or lost previously mailed documents will have a fresh mail-out in hand. It is worthwhile to remember that prospective participants do not center their lives around surveys as do some survey scientists. Within reason, thoughtful actions by the survey team are directed toward one goal: maximize the rate of response to the survey.
- More than 120 trackers were needed to complete the 66,400 screening calls, a task requiring patience, tenacity, and emotional maturity. Given the extraordinary nature of this project, there is no yard stick to determine if the turnover in the number of screeners was excessive or expected. Once contact letters and survey forms were mailed out and completed documents returned to project staff, sharing this news with the phone screeners would have rekindled their motivation.
- The number of initially incorrect addresses was high with 18% of persons on the master SRC list deleted by project staff. The telephone screeners should have diligently called back to resolve doubts about the accuracy of any names or addresses. Such calls may have saved later problems. However, problems rose when stressed trackers had to shout into the phone to make themselves understood by hearing-impaired listeners. In short, phone tracking hard of hearing persons is tedious work requiring attention to details with a low-pay off (1 hit per 66 calls) and is at times stressful. Repeated use of the same phone script makes phone tracking like assembly line work. However, in phone tracking it is hard to see the «final product.»
- Without the resourcefulness and endurance of these phone trackers, this entire project would have been less successful.

Chapter Summary

More than 66,000 telephone calls identified 1,050 hard of hearing persons willing to participate in a follow-up mail survey. Initial contact letters sent to the 1,050 persons determined that 192 persons (18%) were ineligible for reasons such as lacking a correctable name or address. Mailings of survey questionnaires to the remaining 858 persons yielded 313 useable survey forms for the project database. The phone screening exceeded it goal of identifying 1,000 eligible persons.

By contrast, two conditions may have contributed to the modest response to the mail survey. First, the general population is unfamiliar with social research surveys, except for public opinion polling. Second, most hard of hearing persons are uniquely unaccustomed to openly revealing themselves. Morever, numerous examples in the research literature indicate that when consumers with disabilities know about a program or are involved in a multipoint longitudinal study, response rates are usually higher. The University of Arkansas did not have these advantages. Future studies can draw upon the experiences from this first-of-it's-kind project.

The sample was compared to characteristics of hard of hearing persons in the reliable large-scale 1990-91 NHIS. Despite the 36.5% response rate to the mail survey these comparisons determined that the project sample was represented this population for 5 of 8 demographic attributes. Disparities in two comparisons were caused by differences in data collection: the NHIS used household interviews whereas the project used a mail survey. In addition, the obtained sample was generally geographically representative in four broad regions and 37 of the 43 states where mail survey respondents lived. Other data indicated that about 10% of persons in the project sample had more severe hearing loss than those in two other national samples, *thus phone tracking did not under-represent this group*. The information in Tables 5 and 6 was more rigorously tested than that in Table 4 which displayed a larger portion of persons with severe and profound hearing loss. As expected, most individuals in three evaluated samples had a mild to moderate hearing impairment.

Members of the national panel of experts provided the project team with rare expertise. They made the questionnaires more receptive to prospective survey participants, identified major policy areas where applied research was needed, and shared ideas to enhance the later utility of the survey results. It is notable that 70% of the project personnel and advisory panel members had a hearing loss and provided both personal insights and professional adeptness to enhance the success of the project.

This is a first-ever representative national sample with unprecedented in-depth information on the experiences of these adults with employment and vocational rehabilitation. The representativeness of the project sample is a vital requirement so that study results can be generalized, or inferred, to other hard of hearing adults besides those in the obtained sample.

This publication was supported by grant H133G010156 from the National Institute on Disability and Rehabilitation Research, U.S. Department of Education.

PHONE SCREENING QUESTIONS

Hello, I am ___________ calling for the University of Arkansas in Little Rock. We are attempting to locate people who have hearing problems in order to improve services and programs. The University of Arkansas is not selling anything. It will take only a few moments to answer some brief questions. All of your answers will be kept confidential.

If Tdd/Fax Tone Record Telephone Number And Forward To Research And Training Center For Interview.

1. Does anyone in this home have trouble hearing? Yes (GO TO Q2) No (GO TO Q11) Refused (GO TO Q11)
2. . Are you that person?Yes (GO TO Q3) No (GO TO Q3) Refused (GO TO Q11)
3. What is your (or his or her) first name? (USE THIS TO REFER TO PERSON THROUGHOUT INTERVIEW)
   First name provided (GO TO Q6a)
   First name not provided (GO TO Q4)
   Refused (GO TO Q11)
4. If answer to Q2 was Yes, GO TO Q6a.If answer to Q2 was No, ask: Does (NAME OF HEARING-IMPAIRED PERSON) communicate on the phone?
   Yes (ASK TO SPEAK TO PERSON AND GO TO Q6a)
   No (GO TO Q5) Refused (GO TO Q11)
5. Does (NAME OF HEARING-IMPAIRED PERSON) communicate using a teletypewriter or TDD phone?
   Yes (RECORD PHONE NUMBER FOR CALLBACK BY RESEARCH AND TRAINING CENTER AND GO TO Q6a)
   No (GO TO Q6a)
   Refused (GO TO Q11)

6a. We have just a few more questions to ask you or about (NAME OF HEARING-IMPAIRED PERSON).

Without a hearing aid do you or does (NAME OF HEARING-IMPAIRED PERSON) usually have problems in hearing and understanding speech?

Yes (GO TO Q6b)
No (GO TO Q7a)
Not Sure (GO TO Q6b)
Refused (GO TO Q11)

6b. In other words, are you or is (NAME OF HEARING-IMPAIRED PERSON) hard-of-hearing?

Yes (GO TO Q8)
No (GO TO Q7a)
Refused (GO TO Q11)

7a. Without a hearing aid are you or is (NAME OF HEARING-IMPAIRED PERSON) unable to hear and understand speech?

Yes (GO TO Q7b)
Not Sure (GO TO Q7b)
Refused (GO TO Q11)

7b. In other words, are you or is (NAME OF HEARING-IMPAIRED PERSON) deaf?

Yes (GO TO Q8)
Refused (GO TO Q11)

8. In what year were you or (NAME OF HEARING-IMPAIRED PERSON) born?

RECORD YEAR (GO TO Q9)
Refused (GO TO Q11)

9. Are you or is (NAME OF HEARING-IMPAIRED PERSON) presently working, not working, or retired?

Note: Not working includes: homemaker, going to school, too sick to work, do not want a job, cannot find a job.

Working [W] (GO TO Q10)
Not working [NW] (GO TO Q10)
Retired [R] (GO TO Q10)
Refused (GO TO Q11)

10. Faculty with loss of hearing at the University of Arkansas will be conducting a mail survey of Americans like you. The information from the survey will be used only to improve services for hard-of-hearing individuals. All of the information will be kept confidential. Your name will not be reported. Your cooperation with this survey is important. There are no expected risks in participating. You or (NAME OF HEARING-PERSON) are only one of a few persons being asked to participate in this survey. The University of Arkansas wishes to send you or (NAME OF PERSON OF HEARING-IMPAIRED PERSON) a questionnaire in the mail. Would you or (NAME OF PERSON OF HEARING-IMPAIRED PERSON) be willing to volunteer and participate in this mail survey?

Yes (RECORD AND VERIFY FULL NAME AND MAILING ADDRESS. NOTE WORK/RETIREMENT STATUS (Q9) AND INCLUDE PHONE NUMBER (GO TO Q11)
No (GO TO Q11)
Refused (GO TO Q11)
LOOP Q11 MAXIMUM OF THREE TIMES

11. Does anyone else in this home have trouble hearing?

Yes (GO TO Q3)
No (GO TO END)
Refused (GO TO END)
END OF INTERVIEW. That completes my survey. **Thank you for your time**.

References

Adams, P. F., Hendershot, & G. E., Marano, M.A. (1999). Current estimates from the National Health Interview Survey, 1996. *Vital and Health Statistics, 10* (2000). Hyattsville, MD: National Center for Health Statistics.

Arkansas Association of the Deaf. (2000). *Arkansas TTY directory*. Little Rock: Author.

Balsamo, L. M. (In press). Beethoven's secret: The stigma of adult-onset hearing loss. *The Volta Review*.

Benson, V., & Marano, M. A. (1994). Current estimates from the National Health Interview Survey, 1993. *Vital and Health Statistics 10* (190). Hyattsville, MD: National Center for Health Statistics.

Blood, I. M. (1997). The hearing aid effect: Challenges for counseling. *Journal of Rehabilitation, 63* (4), 59-62.

Boone, S., Schroedel, J. G., Watson, D., & Anderson. G. (1996). *Outreach Oklahoma – project C: Consumer needs assessment (Contract report)*. Little Rock: University of Arkansas, Rehabilitation Research and Training Center on Persons who are Deaf or Hard of Hearing.

Bowe, F. G. (1991). National survey on telephone services and products: The views of deaf and hard-of-hearing people. *American Annals of the Deaf, 36* (3), 278-283.

Call, V. R. A., Otto, L. B., & Spenner, K. I. (1982). *Tracking respondents: A multi-method approach*. Lexington, MA: Lexington Books.

Carmen, R. E. (2001). The concept of chi and the resistant patient. *The Hearing Review, 8* (9), 56, 58, 78.

Casanova, G. M., Katkovsky, W., & Hershberger, W. A. (1988). Effects of impaired hearing and favorable vs. unfavorable personal feedback on negative emotional reactions. *Journal of Clinical Psychology, 44* (6), 982-987.

Chartrand, M. S. (2000). The fear of being found out: The dilemma of denial. *The Hearing Review, 7* (3), 72, 74.

Clarridge, B. R., Sheehy, L. S., & Hauser, T. S. (1976). *Tracing members of a panel: A 17-year follow-up* (CDE Working Paper 76-23). Madison: University of Wisconsin, Center for Demography and Ecology.

El-Khiami, A. (1986). Selected characteristics of hearing-impaired rehabilitants of general VR agencies: A sociodemographic profile. In D. Watson, G. Anderson, & M. Taff-Watson (Eds.), *Integrating human resources, technology and systems in deafness*. Silver Spring, MD: American Deafness and Rehabilitation Association.

El-Khiami, A. (1992, June). *Work environments of hard of hearing youth*. A paper presented at the meeting of Self Help for Hard of Hearing People, Cedar Rapids, IA.

El-Khiami, A. (1993). Employment transitions and establishing careers by postsecondary alumni with hearing loss. *The Volta Review, 95* (4) 357-366.

Fowler, F. J. (1984). *Survey research methods*. Beverly Hills, CA: Sage Publications.

Genevie, L. (1988). *Voting intentions during the 1988 election: A comparison of disabled and non-disabled voters*. New York City: Louis Harris and Associates for the National Organization on Disability.

Geyer, P.D., & Schroedel, J.G. (1999a). Conditions influencing the availability of accommodations for workers who are deaf or hard-of-hearing. *Journal of Rehabilitation, 65* (2), 42-50.

Geyer, P.D., & Schroedel, J. G. (1999b). *Influences on job satisfaction for full-time workers with hearing loss* (RT-31 Technical Report). Little Rock: University of Arkansas, Rehabilitation Research and Training Center for Persons who are Deaf or Hard of Hearing.

Goffman, E. (1963). *Stigma: Notes on the management of spoiled identity*. New York: Simon and Schuster.

Harkins, J. E., & Jensema, C. (1988). Needs for sensory devices: An opinion survey. *JADARA, 22* (1), 1-13.

Hetu, R., & Getty, L. (1993). Overcoming difficulties experienced in the work place by employees with occupational hearing loss. *The Volta Review, 95* (4), 391-402.

Hetu, R., Riverin, L., Lalande, N., Getty, L., & St. Cyr, C. (1988). Qualitative analysis of the handicap associated with occupational hearing loss. *British Journal of Audiology,22*, 251-264.

Jaworkski, A., & Stephens, D. (1998). Self-reports on silence as a face-saving strategy by people with hearing impairment. *International Journal of Applied Linguistics, 8* (1), 61-80.

Kagay, M. (1987). *Participation in voting and elections by disabled Americans*. New York City: Louis Harris and Associates for the National Organization on Disability.

Kent, B. A. (2003). Identity issues for hard of hearing adolescents aged 11, 13, and 15 in mainstreamed settings. *Journal of Deaf Studies and Deaf Education, 8* (3), 315-324.

Kerr, P. C., & Cowrie, R. I. D. (1997). Acquired deafness: A multi-dimensional experience. *British Journal of Audiology, 31,* 177-188.

King, D. A., & Thorne, N. R. (1977). *National longitudinal study of the high school class of 1972: Report of third follow-up data collection activities.* Chapel Hill: University of North Carolina, Research Triangle Institute.

Knapp, P. H. (1948). Emotional aspects of hearing loss. *Psychometric Medicine, 10,* 203-222. Cited by Kyle, Jones, & Wood (1985).

Kochkin, S. (1993). Why 20 million in the U.S. don't use hearing aids for their hearing loss. *The Hearing Journal, 46* (1), 20-21, 26-31, 36-37.

Kochkin, S. (1997). MarkeTrak IV: What is the viable market for hearing aids? *The Hearing Journal, 50* (1), 31-38.

Kochkin, S. (2001). The VA and direct mail sales spark growth in hearing aid market. *The Hearing Review, 8* (12), 16, 18, 20, 22, 24, 63-65.

Kyle, J. G., Jones, L. G., & Wood, P .L. (1985). Adjustment to acquired hearing loss: A working model. In H. Orlans (Ed.), *Adjustment to hearing loss* (119-138). San Diego, CA: College-Hill Press.

Kyle, J. G., & Wood, P. (1983). *Social and vocational aspects of acquired hearing loss* (Final report to MSC). Bristol: University of Bristol, School of Education, Centre for Deaf Studies.

Leitman, R., Cooner, E., & Risher, P. (1994). *N.O.D./Harris survey of Americans with disabilities.* New York City: Louis Harris and Associates for the National Organization on Disability.

Lucas, J. W., Schiller, J. S., & Benson, V. (2004). Summary health statistics for U.S. adults: National Health Interview Survey, 2001. *Vital and Health Statistics, 10* (218). Hyattsville, MD: National Center for Health Statistics.

Market Opinion Research. (1989). *The hearing-impaired population of Michigan.* Lansing: Department of Labor, Division on Deafness.

McNeil, J .M. (2000, July). *Employment, earnings, and disability.* Paper presented at the meeting of the Western Economic Association International, Vancouver, British Columbia.

Meadow-Orlans, K. P., & Orlans, H. (1990). Responses to loss of hearing in later life. In D. F. Moores & K. P. Meadow-Orlans (Eds.), *Educational and developmental aspects of deafness.* Washington, D.C.: Gallaudet University Press.

Miller Research Group. (1996). *Oklahoma disability study* (contract final report). Little Rock: University of Arkansas, Department of Rehabilitation Education and Research.

Moore, C. L., & Schroedel, J. G. (2000). *A national profile of the vocational rehabilitation of Americans with hearing loss* (RT-31 Technical Report). Little Rock: University of Arkansas, Rehabilitation Research and Training Center for Persons who are Deaf or Hard of Hearing.

National Center for Health Statistics. (1998). *Current estimates from the National Health Interview Survey, 1995.* [On-line serial]. Available: *www.gov/nchs/faq/disable.* Hyattsville. MD. Author [Producer and distributor].

National Organization on Disability. (2000). *The 2000 N.O.D.-Harris survey of Americans with disabilities.* [On-line]. Available: www.nod.org/hs2000.

Orlans, H., & Meadow-Orlans, K.P. (1984). Who are the members of SHHH? A report on the SHHH questionnaire. *SHHH,5*(5), 3-5.

Pleis, J. R., & Coles, R. (2002). Summary: Health statistics for U.S. adults: National Health Interview survey, 1998. *Vital and Health Statistics, 10* (209). Hyattsville, MD: National Center for Health Statistics.

Ries, P. W. (1985). The demography of hearing loss. In H. Orlans (Ed.), *Adjustment to adult hearing loss* (3-21). San Diego, CA: College-Hill Press.

Ries, P. W. (1994). Prevalence and characteristics of persons with hearing trouble: United States, 1990-91. *Vital and Health Statistics, 10*(188). Hyattsville, MD: National Center for Health Statistics.

Risher, P., & Amorosi, S. (1998). *N.O.D./Harris survey of American with disabilities* (Study No. 828373). Washington, D.C.: National Organization on Disability.

Schein, J. D. (1968). *The deaf community*. Washington, D.C.: Gallaudet College Press.

Schein, J.D. (1996). The demography of deafness. In P. G. Higgins & J. E. Nash (Eds.), *Understanding deafness socially: Continuities in research and theory* (21-43). Springfield, IL: Charles Thomas.

Schein, J. D., & Delk, M. T. (1974). *The deaf population of the United States*. Silver Spring, MD: National Association of the Deaf.

Schein, J. D., Gentile, A., & Haase, K. (1965). Methodological aspects of a hearing ability interview survey. *Vital and Health Statistics, 2* (12). Washington, D.C: U. S. Government Printing Office, 0-787-626.

Scherich, D. L. (1996). Job accommodations in the workplace for persons who are deaf or hard of hearing: Current practices and recommendations. *Journal of Rehabilitation, 62* (April-June), 27-35.

Schroedel, J. G. (1984). Analyzing surveys on deaf adults: Implications for survey research on persons with disabilities. *Social Science and Medicine, 6*, 619-627.

Schroedel, J. G. (1987). Predictors of socioeconomic status. In A. B. Crammatte (Ed.), *Meeting the challenge: Hearing-impaired professionals in the workplace* (93-138). Washington, D.C.: Gallaudet University Press.

Schroedel, J.G., & Geyer, P. D. (1998). *A national profile of the rehabilitation and employment of hard of hearing persons* (RT-31 Technical Report). Little Rock: University of Arkansas, Rehabilitation Research and Training Center for Persons who are Deaf or Hard of Hearing.

Schroedel, J. G., & Geyer, P. D. (2000). Long-term career attainments of deaf and hard of hearing college graduates: Results from a 15-year follow-up survey. *American Annals of the Deaf, 145*(4), 300-311.

Schroedel, J.G., & Geyer, P.D. (2001). Enhancing the career advancement of workers with hearing loss: Results from a national follow-up survey. *Journal of Applied Rehabilitation Counseling, 32* (3), 35-44.

Schroedel, J.G., & Jacobsen, R. J. (1978). *Employer attitudes toward hiring persons with disabilities: A labor market research model* (Report of RSA grant 15-P-59039/2). Albertson, NY: Human Resources Center.

Schroedel, J., Kelley, C., & Conway, P. (2002). Where are all the hard of hearing college students? Some tips for enhancing services by postsecondary and rehabilitation professionals. In K.B. Jursik (Ed.), *Diverse voices, one goal: Conference proceedings* (105-111). Knoxville: University of Tennessee, Postsecondary Education Consortium.

Schroedel, J., Kelley, C., & Conway, P. (2003). *Reaching the «invisible population»: Enhancing vocational rehabilitation and disability support services to hard of hearing college students*. Retrieved November 18, 2003 from Western Oregon University, Western Symposium on the Rehabilitation of the Deaf Website: *http://www.wou.edu/nwoc/wsrd.html.*

Schroedel, J. G., & Watson, D. (1991). *Enhancing opportunities in postsecondary education for deaf students* (Final report of NIDRR grants G008300153 and G0086C3501). Little Rock: University of Arkansas, Rehabilitation Research and Training Center for Persons who are Deaf or Hard of Hearing.

Schroedel, J. G., Watson, D., & Ashmore, D. H. (2005). How many hard of hearing and deaf college students are there? Implications for program planning from a demographic update: A public forum. In K. B. Jursik (Ed.), *Planning for success: Initiatives in positive outcomes – Conference proceedings. Http://sunsite.utk.edu/cod/pec.html.*

Schroedel, J., Watson, D., & Boone, S. (2004, May). *Invigorating VR services to hard of hearing consumers: A processional dialogue on a national research project.* Washington, D.C.: Paper presented at the conference for state coordinators and related professionals serving persons with hearing loss. Retrieved November 23, 2004 from http://www.rcep6.org.

Sorkin, D. L. (1995). Understanding our needs: The SHHH member survey. *SHHH Journal, 16* (2), 22-24.

Sorkin, D. L. (1997). Developing an identity for people with hearing loss. *Hearing Loss, 18* (1), 14-18.

Stika, C. J. (1997). Living with hearing loss -- Focus group results, part II: Career development and work experiences. *Hearing Loss, 18*(6), 29-32.

Stone, D. L., & Colella, A. (1996). A model of factors affecting the treatment of disabled individuals in organizations. *Academy of Management Review, 21* (2), 352-401.

Taylor, H., Kagay, M. R., & Leichenko, S. (1986). *The ICD survey of disabled Americans: Bringing disabled Americans into the mainstream.* New York: Louis Harris and Associates.

Taylor, H., & Wurf, N. (1991). *Public attitudes toward people with disabilities.* New York City: Louis Harris and Associates for the National Organization on Disability.

TDI. (2001). *The blue book: National directory and resources guide.* Silver Spring, MD: Author.

Thomas, A., Lamont, M., & Harris, M. (1982). Problems encountered at work by people with severe acquired hearing loss. *British Journal of Audiology, 16*, 39-43.

Tomlinson, P. A. (1992). *Rehabilitation of individuals who are hard of hearing and late deafened: A guide for administrators.* Hot Springs: University of Arkansas, Region VI Rehabilitation Continuing Education Program.

Trupin, M. P. H., Sebesta, D. S., Yelin, E., & La Plante, M. P. (1997). *Trends in labor force participation among persons with disabilities, 1983-1994.* San Francisco: University of California, Disability Statistics Rehabilitation Research and Training Center.

Trybus, R., Stika, C., & Goulder, J. (2004). *Maintaining employment status and enhancing personal adjustment for people with hearing loss* (Report of NIDRR grant HI33840022). San Diego: California School of Professional Psychology, Rehabilitation Research and Training Center on Individuals who are Late-Deafened or Hard of Hearing.

U.S. Census Bureau. (1999). *Statistical abstract of the United States* (119th ed.). Austin, TX: Hoover's Business Press.

U.S. Census Bureau. (2003). *Statistical abstract of the United States* (123rd ed.). Austin, TX: Hoover's Business Press.

U.S. Commission on Civil Rights. (1998). *Helping employers comply with the ADA*. Washington, DC: U. S. Government Printing Office 1998-444-783/90797.

Weinstein, B. E. (1996). Treatment efficacy: Hearing aids in the management of hearing loss in adults. *Journal of Speech and Hearing Research, 39*(5), s37-s45.

INDEX

C

D

E

F

G

H

I

N

O

P

Q

R

S

T

U

V

W

Y